The Beauty Workbook

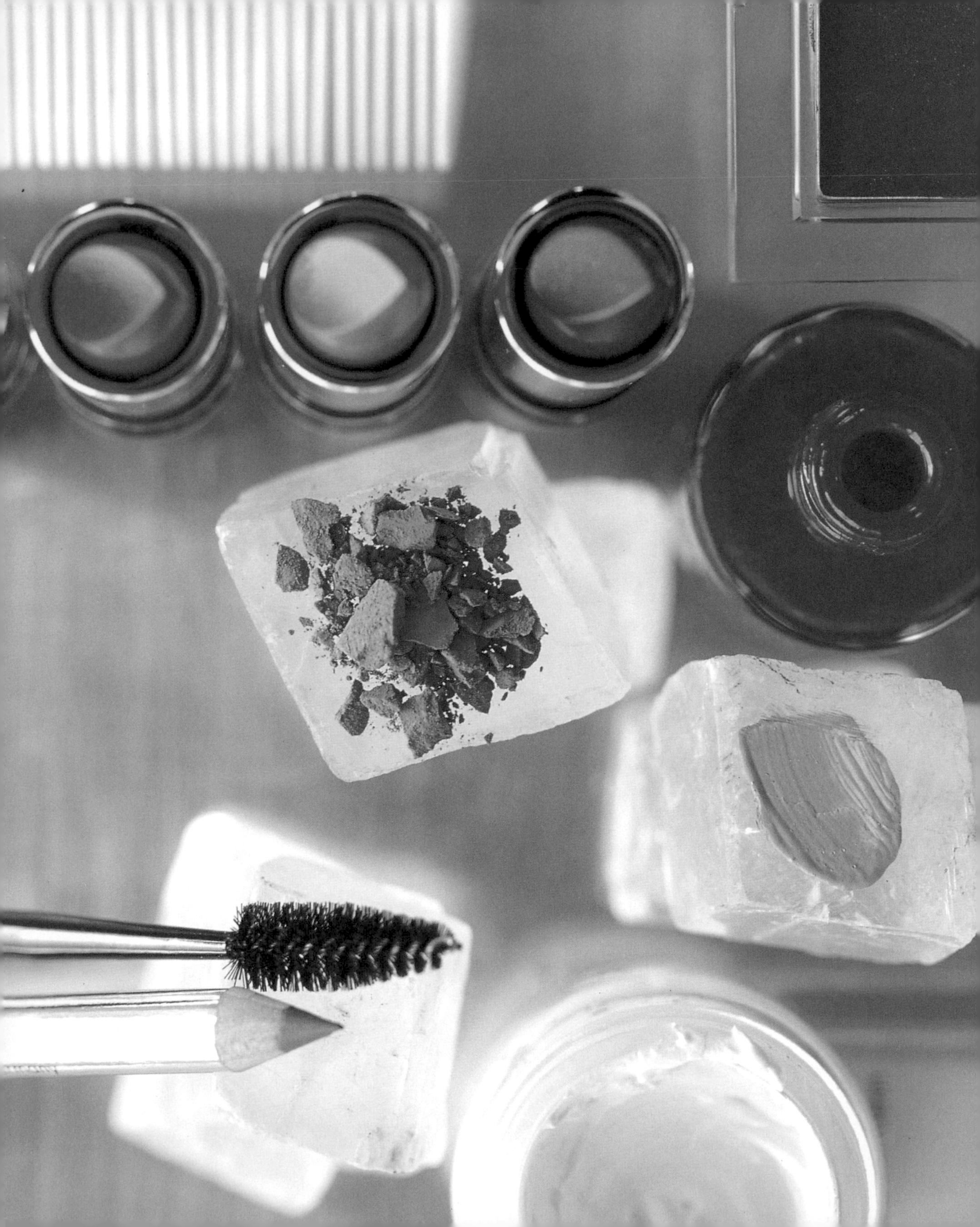

The Beauty Workbook

A Commonsense Approach
to Skin Care, Makeup, Hair, and Nails

By Cynthia Robins

Photographs by Laurie Frankel

Illustrations by Kelly Burke

CHRONICLE BOOKS
SAN FRANCISCO

To Ron Pernell, my dear friend and creator of beauty and dreams.

To every makeup artist I've ever learned anything from.

To the memory of my elegant and proper mother, Rhoda Shore, who taught me to use moisturizer when I was a tender teen.

And finally, to the memory of my dapper, handsome, youthful father, Jack Shore, who gifted me with his glorious Russian genes.

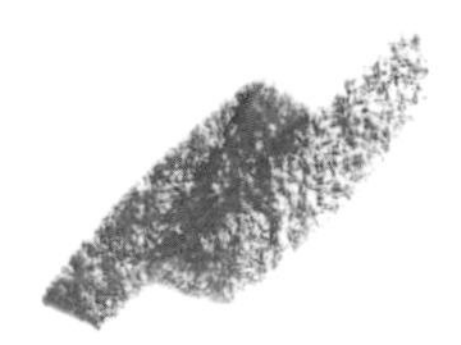

Library of Congress Cataloging-in-Publication Data available.

ISBN: 0-8118-2385-7

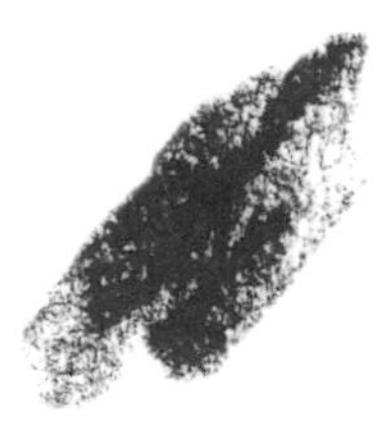

Printed in Hong Kong
Designed by Laurie Frankel
Styling by Julie Muszynski
Typeset in Joanna MT and Lubalin Graph

Distributed in Canada by Raincoast Books
9050 Shaughnessy Street
Vancouver, British Columbia V6P 6E5

10 9 8 7 6 5 4 3 2

Chronicle Books LLC
85 Second Street
San Francisco, California 94105
www.chroniclebooks.com

table of contents

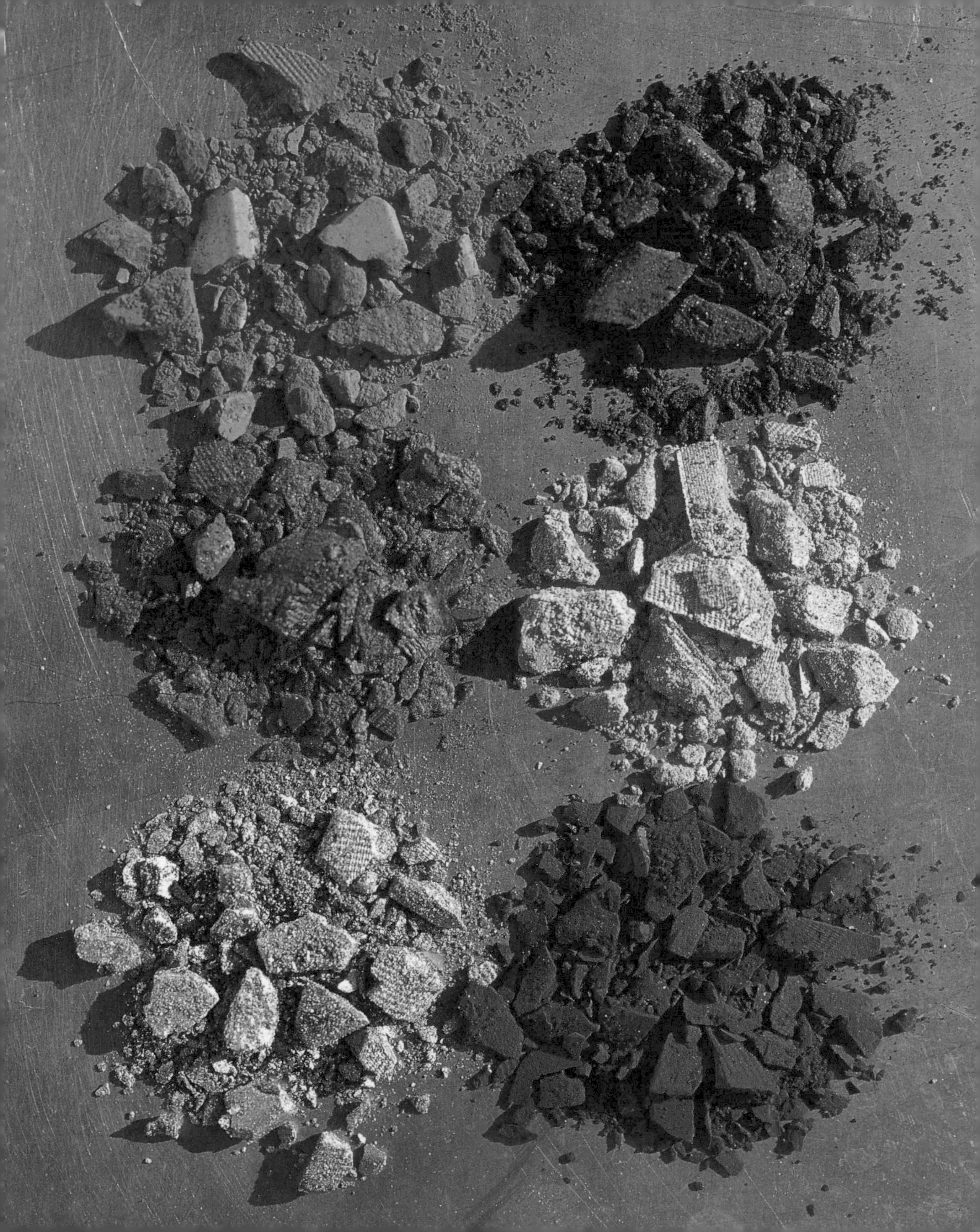

INTRODUCTION

Have you ever strolled through the cosmetics department of a major department store and become so confused by the myriad of choices that you simply left? You are not alone. There are many women—lovely, accomplished, grown-up, fearless, *complete* women—who feel so undone by the thousands of products offered by the hundreds of cosmetics companies beckoning to them, like Eve with her shiny apple, that they simply refuse to engage. The vast array of care and color options is overwhelming, even intimidating. There are lipsticks, mascaras, eyeshadows, powders, and blushers, soaps, scrubs, sprays, eye gels, lip balms, pore tighteners, moisturizers, masks, and miracle creams, not to mention the constant barrage of advertisements and editorial opinions in slick women's magazines, newspaper beauty columns, and Web sites.

A girl could drown in a sea of promises. "Use me!" tempts a slick ad featuring a smooth-faced woman who has probably never known a blemish in her life (or who has, more realistically, been airbrushed into perfection), and you, even *you*, can have smoother, clearer, more inviting skin. You, too, can look younger. Be more enticing. Live the same life as our enchantingly gorgeous model. The hype—albeit written in glowing terms with hopeful phrases like *promotes a youthful appearance, reduces visible signs of aging, returns the glow of youth*—is simply that. Just hype. Designed to get you interested enough to spend $10 or $80 for a little bit of cream in a jar that promises everything but delivers nothing.

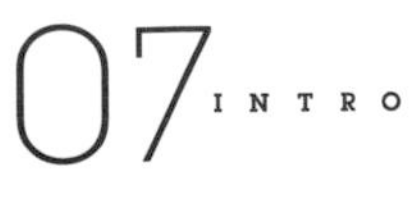

Couple the intimidation factor of waltzing through a virtual cosmetic circus where vitrines glitter with inviting arrays of artfully packaged product, with the image of a 19-year-old model advertising a skin preparation for 40-year-olds, and one of three things can happen. You can decide to play and leave the store loaded down with product you don't need and haven't a clue how to use. Or, you can exhibit a natural fear response and think: "Oh, dear, I must be inadequate, less than a woman. I cannot choose. Think I'll just go home." Or, you can aggressively shun those things you deem feminine by refusing to take part: "I'm not the makeup type. Besides, with my [fill in the blank here: family, career, personal] obligations, who has time for all this froufrou anyhow? Forget about it."

We women have each been given one face, one skin type, and an entire lifetime to mess it up. We use harsh detergent soaps on our faces, which strip natural oils from our skin; we take baths in extra-hot water and wonder why we flake and itch. We go to the gym in full face-paint, sweat like stevedores, then want to know why we're breaking out. And after we've spent our teen years basted in baby oil tinted with Mercurochrome, flipping periodically like burgers on the barbecue, we learn that the little growth near our nose is a skin cancer.

All that product, all those potential problem solvers in jars, tubes, and bottles, all that knowledge swirling around in one huge informational soup that has become too complicated to cope with and too time consuming to take advantage of—it is a dilemma, isn't it? And yet, as we age and our faces begin to reflect what years, gravity, the environment, and just plain indifference have wrought, decoding the mythos of cosmetics and skincare becomes not a vanity or a luxury but a virtue and a necessity.

The Beauty Workbook will help to remove the overlay of self-criticism, confusion, and neglect from what can be feminine and nurturing, as well as just plain frivolous good fun. At some point, the mirror does not lie. (Well, it never did, did it?) And most women—from working women or high-profile careerists to devoted mothers to those who have chosen to follow multiple paths—eventually realize that they have not paid enough attention to themselves. In their traditional role as mother and nurturer, or in the contemporary role of overscheduled, overstimulated, overaggressive business or career woman, the last person they take care of (or reward) during their days of tending to the needs and demands of others is themselves.

The Beauty Workbook lobbies for taking the time to care for what nature has provided. It is a celebration of femaleness for all shapes, sizes, ages, and colors. Here you will find basic hands-on how-to information about commonsense skincare and makeup. Take *The Beauty Workbook* into the bathroom and use it like a cookbook. Slip it into your tote or backpack and take it to the cosmetic counter.

In *The Beauty Workbook*, you'll find a handy pocket to store pamphlets, newspaper clips, and magazine articles about new developments and products you'd like to try. And there are thought-provoking, imagination-stimulating questionnaires and exercises that place the focus directly on you, your misconceptions, your hopes, your dreams, your fantasies.

But most of all, *The Beauty Workbook* is designed to take the hocus-pocus and confusion out of the basics of skincare, makeup, and sun, hair, and nail care. You'll learn about the physical composition of your skin, how we age, and how common sense and a simple regimen can slow the aging process and correct many of the ravages of sun exposure and environmental pollution. You'll get the very simple basics of makeup—quick-trick solutions that work on every face shape and skin type.

But before it's time to contemplate lipstick, blusher, eye shadow, and powder, you have to get your complexion into shape. Makeup artists are fond of referring to faces as "blank canvases." And as for any artist, the canvas must be prepared before the art of beauty can begin.

This preparation starts from within with a proper diet of fresh fruits and vegetables, whole grains, protein, and water. Lots and lots of water. So much water that sometimes you feel like you're drowning in it. Your skin will respond to commonsense practices: eating well, drinking plenty of water,

and getting enough exercise and sleep. Your body uses its downtime to rest and repair. When your metabolism slows, the rejuvenation process has an opportunity to work. New skin cells are born; old ones slough off on your pillow. And in the morning, after you've cleaned the sleep grit and oil from your face, you can stand in front of your mirror and decide who you want to be.

The Beauty Workbook is for women who want to look finished but not "done." It is for those who can't, won't, or shouldn't take more than 10 minutes with their makeup. It offers you a basic primer for modernizing your look with a minimum of fuss and ways to do so in as little time as possible. Colors exist in new cosmetic formulas that go on easily and last the whole day. Quick and easy application can make the difference between a dated face that is fixed in time (like the woman who clings to her blonde Farrah Fawcett wings and beige lipstick of the 1970s because that's how she remembers feeling her best) and a look that is fresh and contemporary.

The Beauty Workbook is not designed to give you 15 ways to do your eyes. Rather, it explains the basis of good makeup technique—starting with eyebrows that frame the face and ending with a fluff of powder, a splash of scent, a smile to the mirror, and a confident stroll out the door.

Add to that the finishing touches of healthy hair and no-nonsense, strong, and attractive nails, and you have *The Beauty Workbook*—truly a commonsense approach to the age-old tradition of feminine beauty.

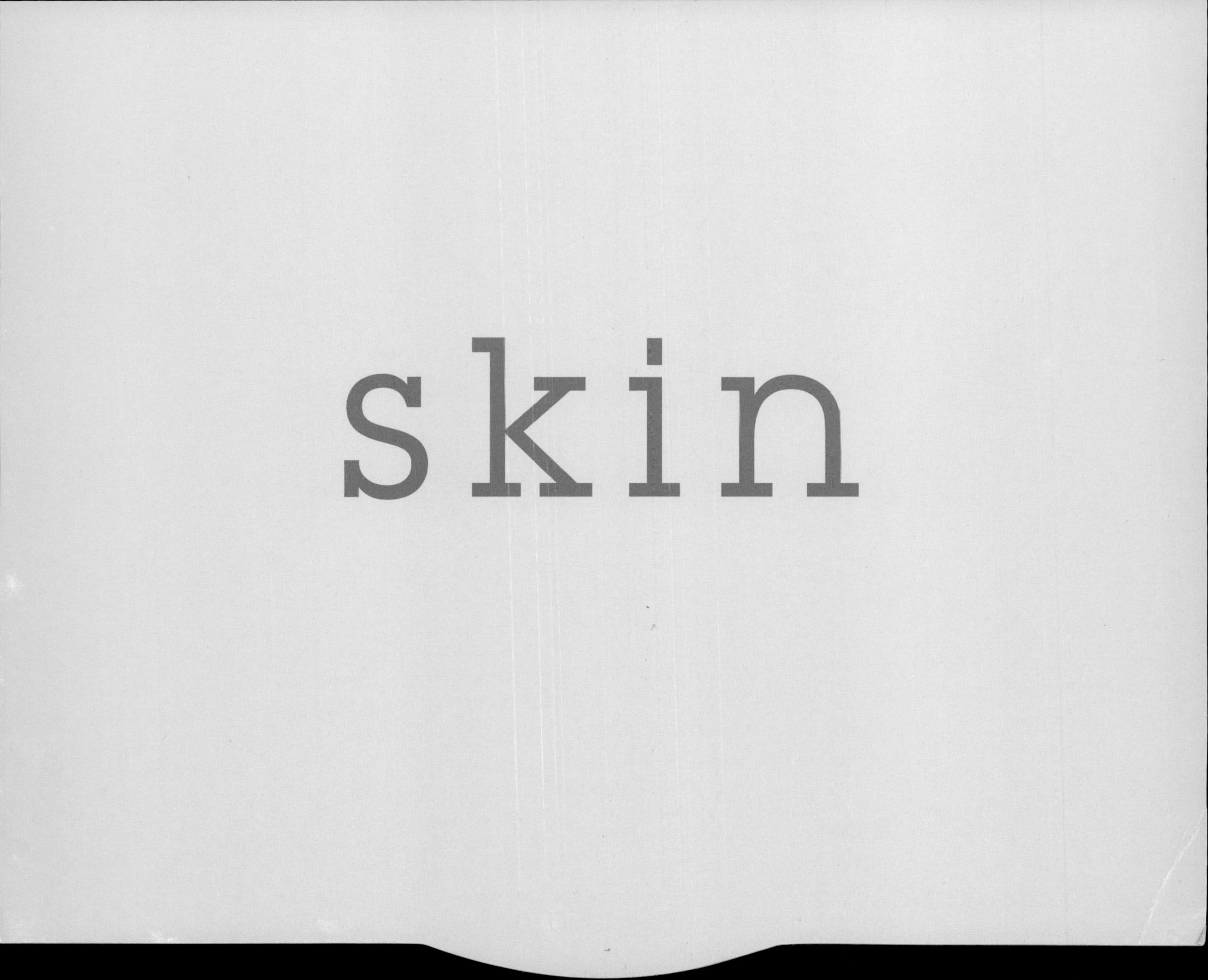
skin

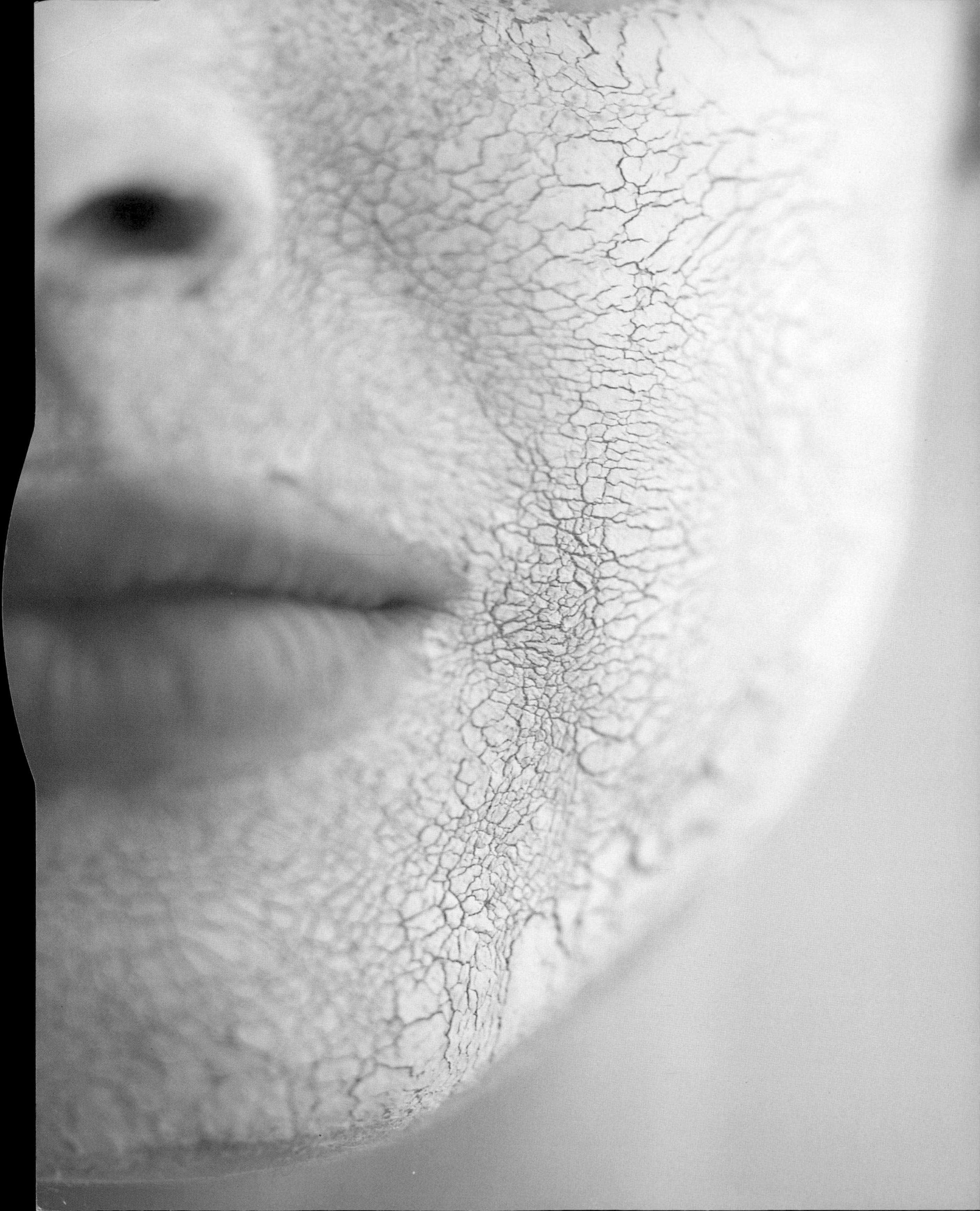

CHAPTER ONE: SKIN

Consider it the cosmetic Dark Age, but way back in 1958, when Charles Revson, founder of Revlon, held up a jar of his latest skin cream, Eterna 27, and said, "This is hope in a jar," he was selling fantasy and playing on women's worst fears—that someday they would be old and no longer beautiful. His implied promise was: Use this product and you will remain young (read: *beautiful*) and forever appear under 30. In reality, Revson was selling not only hope, but also hype in a jar. His new brand of moisturizer made the kinds of claims women have clung to. It was no better, and certainly no worse, than anything else on the market at the time.

Ever since, we've been looking for the Fountain of Youth at the cosmetic counter. We spend untold millions, no make that billions, of dollars yearly on potions, lotions, salves, gels, and creams in the hope of slowing or reversing the wrinkles and lines of time. Here's the real skinny: There is no magic bullet or miracle cream. You cannot turn back the clock or undo what years of gravity, indifference, sun exposure, and environmental pollutants have done to your skin—unless, of course, you have an intimate and ongoing relationship with your plastic surgeon. For most women, plastic surgery is a scary, expensive, and unacceptable option.

So what is the alternative?

For older women who may have done untold harm to their skin in their youth, there is proof that some of the damage is reversible—through physician-assisted chemical peels or laser resurfacing, or more gradually using newly developed over-the-counter exfoliating agents, antioxidants, and a new category of products, which the industry calls *cosmeceuticals,* or cosmetics that produce a mild drug reaction on a cellular level. (Because of FDA regulations, cosmetic companies cannot advertise the full potential of their new products. Therefore, advertising claims are more oblique than direct, with such wording as: *produces the appearance of younger skin* or *helps the skin's ability to retain moisture.*)

For your teenaged daughters, however, knowledge *is* the Fountain of Youth. Forewarned is forearmed. The message mothers should be giving their daughters, along with a good sunscreen, is: Take good care of the skin you were born with; you cannot replace it.

Sometimes I wish I had never seen the sun. Like the day a dermatologist removed a precancerous growth from my face and said: "You were a sun bunny, weren't you?" He saw the evidence of the summers of my youth, a halcyon idyll of sunny days misspent, slathered in baby oil dosed with iodine, like so much marinade. The goal: a deep, dark tan.

We stroked on the oil, stretched out by the pool (with the sun caroming off both water and concrete), and set an oven timer to 15 minutes. When the bell rang, we flipped like trout in a pan. So we got sunburned. So we peeled. Some of us even blistered and endured sleepless nights. But we were dark teenaged goddesses with the tan lines to prove it. Now, as older women, we pay the toll with teensy lines, lack of elasticity, dryness, discoloration, and cancerous growths. At 35 and 40, the porcelain skin we were born with is just a happy memory. The fees for youthful indiscretion in the sun always get collected many years later. You might think: *Now they tell me.* It means little when you realize that most of the effects of the sun—called "photo aging"—could have been prevented.

The question is: What can we do about it now? Revson held up his "hope in a jar" at the same time the Russians fired off Sputnik, the first vehicle in space. Today, far into the space age, there are modern formulations released through high-tech delivery systems that work with such penetrating action that they can actually affect the skin on a cellular level. Many are called "miracle creams"—the alpha- and beta-hydroxy acids (AHAs and BHAs), the retinols, the serums of vitamin C or E, the cosmeceuticals—and with regular and carefully controlled use, they can make a difference in the appearance of your skin. Couple these formulations with proper eating habits; more water than you thought you could ever drink; the elimination of alcohol, tobacco, and caffeine; and an excellent sunblock applied liberally to your face, neck, and hands every day, and maybe, just maybe, it is possible to regain some of what age and the environment have taken from you.

It's important to understand exactly what your skin is, how it works to protect you, and how it ages.

But before we get to a discussion of true hope in a jar, it's important to understand exactly what your skin is, how it works to protect you, and how it ages.

THE ORGAN RECITAL

Your skin is the one organ that is brazen enough to appear naked in public. It's the largest organ of your body, encompassing 20 square feet were it laid out like a carpet, and weighing between 7 and 9 pounds. Skin is the most flexible organ, even more so than the heart; it is also the most versatile, performing numerous functions.

Imagine that your skin is a huge, waterproof, leakproof but permeable, super-stretchable sack that keeps your insides in and the environment and germs out. Skin is your own personal all-weather gear. It is all that comes between you and the outside world. Therefore, it is subject to heat, cold, rain, bacteria, sun, and chemical and environmental pollution. Cushioning your inner organs like a layer of bubble wrap, it is your largest erogenous zone, responsive to touch and temperature.

Your skin is a barometer of your emotions, your personality, and your general health. It is often one of the first indicators that something is amiss in your body. For instance, yellow (or, jaundiced) skin means a change in kidney or liver function. A pimple? That is usually an immediate reflection of your stress level, your dietary habits, or pollution.

Your facial skin, the most tender and vulnerable, is also a mirror of how well you have cared for yourself. Unless you have had plastic surgery or laser resurfacing, your skin will not hide careless disregard for your own best interests. If you smoke, take drugs, drink excessive amounts of alcohol, or expose yourself, unprotected, to sunshine, your skin will never lie.

When we are born, our skin is the best it will ever be: flawless, smooth, pure, refined, sheer, translucent like fine porcelain. Throughout our lifetime, it is our first line of defense, our permeable but protective armor. The miracle of skin is that is it constantly renewing and replenishing itself.

A cross section of skin reveals many layers, each one performing a distinct function. One layer produces new, healthy skin cells; another layer is for the development of spongy proteins, called collagen and elastin, that support the skin like bedsprings. And yet another layer is where hair follicles originate and where subcutaneous fat cushions the entire structure. On the surface, your skin looks pretty placid, but for each ½-inch-square section of it, there are 100 sweat glands, at least 10 hairs, more than 3 feet of capillaries, and 15 oil glands.

The Epidermis

The very top of the epidermis—the part of the skin that gets all of the abuse and receives most of the pleasure—is called the *stratum corneum*. Comprising four or five microscopic layers and as thick as a piece of Xerox paper, under magnification it looks like a shingled roof composed of millions of spent skin cells. Individually, the cells are flattened husks of protein called *keratin*. They are linked together by a chemical bond, and they slough off when you wash your face, rub your skin with a towel or washcloth, or burrow into your pillowcase. We lose exhausted skin cells all the time—30 percent of household dust is really dead skin cells.

Skin cells are formed in the bottom of the epidermis and take three weeks to wander to the surface and slough off. In aging skin, the trip upward can take longer and the process becomes less orderly. Cells aren't as neat and tidy and don't exfoliate quickly. Groups of spent skin cells that appear patchy and dull have lost the ability to move in an orderly, prescheduled fashion. Professional facials, papaya masks, or the regular use of a commercial exfoliant, such as an AHA (which will chemically break up the glue holding the cells together), accelerate the process. Freshly cleaned or exfoliated skin glows because the dead keratin has been flushed away.

The bottom layer of the epidermis, the basal layer, contains melanocytes, which produce melanin, the dark brown pigment that gives skin its color. Everyone has the same number of melanocytes, but the depth of color developed in the melanin is determined by genetic heritage. Melanin is nature's way of protecting the skin from the ultraviolet rays of the sun. When we tan, our melanin has been stimulated to produce a natural barrier to invading sunlight.

The Dermis

A subepidermal layer of skin, the dermis, produces protein fibers called *collagen* and *elastin*—the skin's natural box springs. Healthy, young collagen fibers stand up straight; the skin looks plump and springs back immediately when you touch it. The erosive and destructive properties of the sun, tobacco smoke, alcohol, drugs, and time itself twist, shrivel, and beat the fibers down into flattened mats. Where the skin's support system has been compromised, gullies, rivulets, and indentations can appear on the surface in the form of fine lines and wrinkles.

The dermis is dense with sweat and sebaceous glands, blood vessels, hair follicles, and nerves. A single human being has 2 to 5 million sweat glands snaking through the dermis, opening up as pores in the stratum corneum. Sweat glands are nature's thermostat; they regulate body temperature by expelling impurities, water, and salt.

The skin's natural humectant is *sebum*, or sebaceous oil. Slightly acidic, sebum forms the protective mantle on the skin's surface, lubricating it, keeping it soft, and shutting out harmful bacteria. You can strip the natural oils from your skin with overuse of harsh detergent soaps, abrasive scrubs, sticky pore strips, or granular masks with large, irregular particles (almond and salt scrubs are the bad guys here). Without sebum's protective mantle, your skin is subject to irritation, redness, and chapping.

The Subcutaneous Fatty Layer

Underlying both the dermis and the epidermis is a subcutaneous fatty layer that stores fat cells and strands of collagen and connective tissue. It is the skin's natural shock absorber, which protects and cushions inner organs and helps support the skin. The fatty layer stores nutrients and retains heat. Nerves and blood vessels meander through it. Women have more subcutaneous fat than men, which gives their skin a lustrous resiliency that men do not have.

The miracle of nature is that skin can take a whole lot of abuse and still perform the functions for which it was designed. But since your skin meets the outside world, sometimes the damage inflicted on it by nature, compounded by genetic predetermination and the dilatory effects of self-inflicted abuse (sun, alcohol, tobacco, pharmaceuticals), ages you prematurely. A 35-year-old who spent her youth waterskiing or playing tennis without proper sun protection can look older than a 50-year-old who has lived under long sleeves, sunscreen, and a hat.

The Genetic Gift: Determining Your Skin Type

If there were no sun, chemicals, or bacteria, no martinis, merlot, or Miller beer, your skin would probably do what it was meant to do—that is, what your genetic plot has predetermined. Genes determine how our skin behaves and ages. But wouldn't it be nice if you could push a button or take a pill and change the color or texture of your skin at will? That is not possible. Our genes are our destiny, and we must learn to live with both their gifts and their jokes.

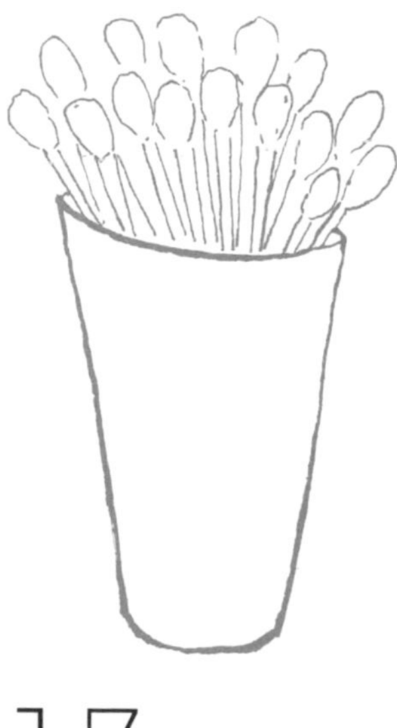

Our genes are our destiny, and we must learn to live with both their gifts and their jokes.

Skin-Type Determination Quiz

1. **When I'm out in the sun, does my skin burn, peel, and then tan?**
2. **After I cleanse my skin, does it feel tight and tingly? Itchy?**
3. **Does my face feel like a puddle of oil an hour after I've washed it? Does my makeup disappear by midmorning? At age 30, am I still breaking out like a teenager?**
4. **Does my skin feel as tight as a drum when I wash in hot water? Does it reflect light, or does it appear dull and patchy? Can I see flakes or red spots where there used to be clear skin?**

Interpretation

If you answered yes to question 1, chances are your skin is dry or sensitive. If you said yes to question 2, your skin is most likely combination—normal in some places, oily in others. If you said yes to question 3, you have oily skin with overactive sebaceous glands. If you said yes to question 4, your skin is aging.

ONE OF FIVE

Dermatologists usually type healthy, normal skin in five categories: normal/combination, dry, oily, sensitive, and aging.

1. Normal/Combination Skin: This is skin that maintains a healthy balance. With combination skin, you can have two kinds of skin at the same time. Your cheeks can be neither dry nor oily, but your T-zone—the area formed by forehead, nose, and chin—can be a little oily. Often the pores around your nose are larger than those on the rest of your face. With sun exposure, you'll probably burn the first time out but the burn will turn to tan quickly. You'll break out occasionally, but by and large you've passed that stage by your 20s, and your skin will behave quite nicely under non-stressful situations. As you age, fine lines will appear around your eyes, forehead, and lips.

2. Dry skin: Yours is thinner, paler skin that burns easily in the sun and feels itchy when the temperature gets colder. After you've cleansed, your skin feels tight and tingly, and in cold weather, you can see raised welts and white lines where you've "drawn" on your skin. Your skin will probably flake in cold weather or after a hot bath if you do not protect it with creams and moisturizers.

Dry skin is dehydrated skin; moisture has taken a permanent vacation. Affected by changes in season, hot water, prescription medications, recreational drugs, alcohol, cigarettes, sun exposure, or air travel (there is nothing worse for any kind of skin than the recycled, canned air in planes), dry skin sheds skin cells in clumps and looks scaly or red.

3. Oily skin: If you are among the 60 percent of women who still get pimples and blackheads in their 30s and 40s, you most likely have oily skin. Oily skin has more melanin and can be darker in tone; you tan with sun exposure and rarely burn. You also have ultra-active sebaceous glands and larger pores. If, for instance, your face is covered with a light sheen of oil an hour after cleansing, or if your makeup seems to sink into your skin before noon, you have oily skin.

4. Sensitive skin: The cause of sensitive skin is a weak protective lipid barrier. Lipids are fatty molecules that lock moisture in the surface of the skin and guard against temperature extremes and environmental pollutants. It seems as if everything negative that can occur with skin happens to sensitive skin types. You burn with sun exposure. You get allergic reactions to food, pollen, soap, chemicals in drinking water, fragrances, and other irritants and break out, turn red and blotchy, or feel itchy, tight, and uncomfortable.

Where new cell turnover used to take two to three weeks, it now takes a month or more for cells to migrate from the basal layer to the skin surface.

You need sun protection the most, but the irony is that chemical sunscreens and sunblocks with the proper sun protection will probably occlude your pores and cause blackheads and breakouts.

If you've had sensitive, allergic skin your whole life, you know what causes your breakouts. Avoid scrubs and abrasive puffs, which are anathema to sensitive skin, as is regular use and overuse of exfoliants such as AHAs and BHAs, or tretinoin acid (the active ingredient in prescription Retin-A and over-the-counter retinol products). Sensitive skin can get dry and patchy and calls for gentle exfoliation once in a while, but abuse of any exfoliants will further destroy the guardian lipid barrier.

5. Aging skin: As we age, our metabolism and circulation slow, which means less oxygen is available to carry nutrients to the skin. As cell renewal slows, the regular, cyclical process of cell regeneration and exfoliation isn't as neat and tidy as it once was. Where new cell turnover used to take two to three weeks, it now takes a month or more for cells to migrate from the basal layer to the skin surface. So your skin does not look or feel as smooth; there is a loss of radiance as dead skin cells clump and refract light unevenly. Meanwhile, melanin-bearing cells thin out and grow less efficient. The sun follies of youth have served to dry out the skin, which is getting loose, saggy, blotched, and discolored with sun spots and freckles. Photo aging produces leathery, ultra-dry skin, broken blood vessels, and *actinic keratoses*, or precancerous growths.

In aging skin we can see the damage caused by rogue oxygen ions called *free radicals*, which are the by-products of sun exposure, alcohol and tobacco use, and environmental pollution. Proper oxygen molecules have two oxygen ions; free radicals have only one and are constantly looking to disrupt healthy O_2 molecules by trying to pair up. In metal, free radicals cause rust. In human beings, they disrupt a healthy cell's ability to manufacture proteins and divide. The abnormal proteins formed by free radicals can produce mutant cells and malignancies.

During menopause, skin goes through noticeable changes. The pores by your nose enlarge. Skin thins out, becomes dull and less light reflective. Estrogen levels are reduced by half to two-thirds at the onset of menopause, so taking hormones may be indicated as a way of slowing the aging process. With HRT (hormone replacement therapy), skin can regain some of its ability to retain moisture and suppleness, but that extra influx of estrogen causes other problems. Hot flashes come with menopause. They are your body's attempt to adjust to fluctuating estrogen levels that blotch and blush your skin. Pimples, whiteheads, and blackheads appear where they never did before.

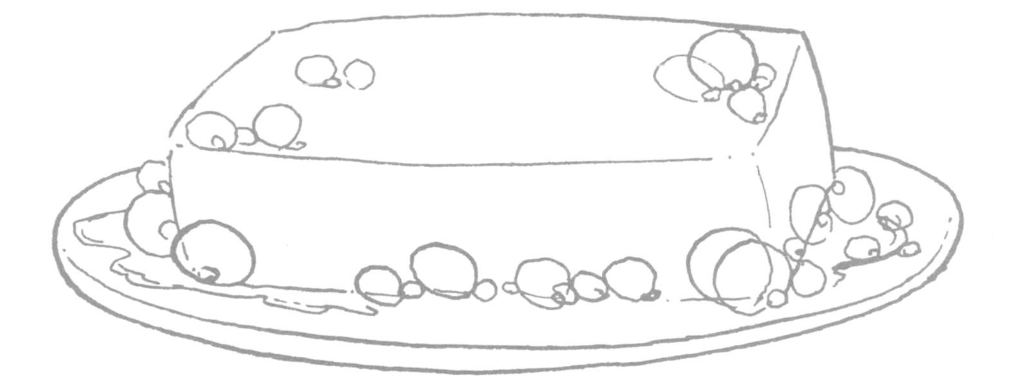

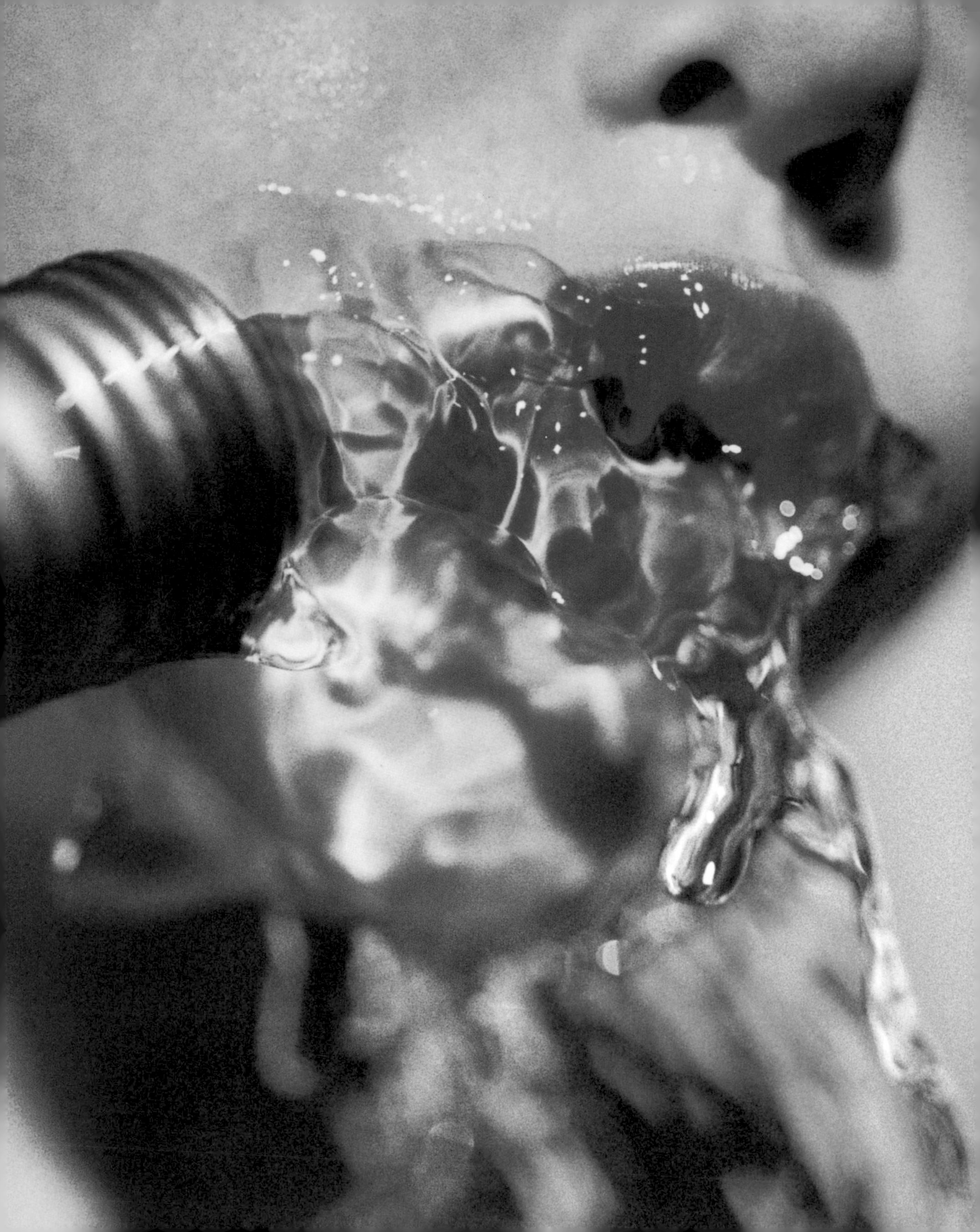

CARING ENOUGH TO TAKE GOOD CARE

We are all born with skin that is affected by our genetic maps, but we still have choices. We can ignore what nature has presented us with and treat our skin poorly by pulling, scratching, stretching, or abrading it. We can continue to abuse it by indulging in too much sun, alcohol, drugs, and caffeine. Or we can be alert, careful, and loving toward our skin.

Each skin type requires both general and specific attention to look its best. The following steps can work for all skin types:

- **Drink water**—a lot of water. In fact, the importance of water intake cannot be stressed enough. By drinking a minimum of eight 8-ounce glasses of water a day, you can actually make a visible difference in your skin in about two weeks. Your skin glows with health when you drink water. Water is both a hydrating and a cleansing agent; it forces evaporation. Drink it in and wash toxins and waste products out—either by perspiration and evaporation through the pores or by urination. The result: finer textured skin, what aestheticians call clarity and radiance.
- **Cut down your caffeine.** Limit yourself to a single cup of tea or coffee or change your Earl Gray to a decaf or herbal variety. (Herbal teas count as part of your daily water intake. Hooray!) Caffeine, like alcohol, is a diuretic and will dry your skin.
- **Stop smoking.** Smoke, tars, nicotine—all are drying agents and contain carcinogens. Warning labels on cigarette packs caution that smoking causes heart problems, lung cancer, and pregnancy complications. What they don't list is skin damage.
- **Protect yourself in the sun** and limit your overall exposure. One out of every seven Americans will develop some form of skin cancer. Be aggressive in protecting yourself from the sun. A little bit is very good for us, but a glass of orange juice will give you the same vitamin D benefits as 10 minutes in the sun (which is the

recommended daily requirement). Never leave home without some kind of sunscreen on your face with an SPF (sun protection factor) of at least 15. Cosmetic companies are developing moisturizers and foundations with SPFs in them. Use them. Put sunscreen on your hands, on the back of your neck, in your part line, and on your ears. Even on cloudy days, the long rays of the sun can penetrate clouds, fog, auto glass, and even 9 feet of water.

CARING FOR YOUR SKIN, TYPE BY TYPE

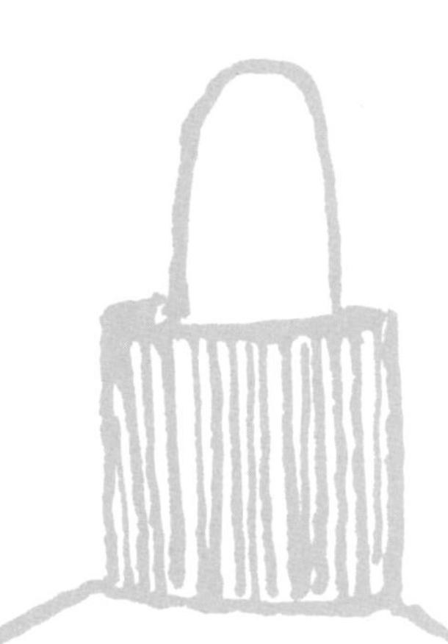

Care of Normal/Combination Skin

Less is more. Your skin is already in balance and the less you do to it in the way of scrubs, toners with alcohol, hot-water cleansing, and detergent soaps, the more it will behave. Cleanse with mild soap and tepid water or with a water-soluble lotion or cream that rinses off. Limit toner use and choose one that is alcohol free and won't disturb the skin's protective mantle. Pat dry with a clean fluffy towel and protect immediately, while your skin is still damp, with a light film of moisturizer. Before you go out in the world—as regularly as brushing your teeth—use sunscreen.

Once a week, give your face a treat—a home facial with a papaya enzyme mask or an exfoliation. Do not expect miracles to happen overnight. AHAs and second-generation exfoliants, BHAs (beta-hydroxy acids), work slowly, but overuse will dry your skin and cause it to blotch and turn red. Have patience, because it will be at least a month before you see some difference.

Care of Dry Skin

Cleanse dry skin with tepid water and a nondetergent soap; detergent soaps strip natural oils. Stay away from hot water, which makes your skin lose moisture through fast evaporation. Stick to rinse-off lotions or cream cleansers or nonsoaps. Moisturize when your skin is still a little damp to lock in your skin's own natural moisture. Dry skin can benefit from a moisture boost at night, so choose a night cream that has a little more weight and contains moisture-keepers called humectants. Look for noncomedogenic creams, or creams that will not clog pores.

Even dry skin needs regular exfoliation. Dry skin can stand limited AHA use, but only once every two weeks. Most dry skin has suffered sun damage, and a dermatologist could suggest using a prescription vitamin A product to retexture the surface of your skin. Retin-A, the prescription form of tretinoin acid, or vitamin A, is very strong and drying; it thins the skin and makes it much more sun sensitive. Retin-A and Renova, two products available only from your doctor, should be used only in the prescribed dosage. There are, however, over-the-counter skin products available in all price ranges that contain retinol, a commercial derivative of tretinoin, which is much milder and works more slowly. Use good sense and moderation with these products.

Care of Oily Skin

Like women with normal/combination skin, those with oily skin should use a minimalist approach. Let's not get overzealous about scrubbing our faces or using cotton balls sopped with harsh, oil-stripping toners and astringents. They'll only inspire already overactive sebaceous glands to pump out even more oil, as skin will send out the wrong message (*Help me, I'm too dry*). Oil production is stimulated by alcohol, spicy foods, and iodines in shellfish as well as overcleansing. Common sense says that if you have oily skin, don't touch your face with dirty hands. (Don't touch your face, period, regardless of what skin type you have). Don't exercise with makeup on. Trade your telephone handset for a headset.

Even the oiliest skin needs moisturizer and rehydration. Look for an oil-free moisturizer. Here is where sampling at the cosmetic counter comes in handy. Before you commit to a product that could block your pores or cause breakouts, get a three-day sample and observe its effects carefully. If you like the way it smells, feels, and reacts on your skin, buy it.

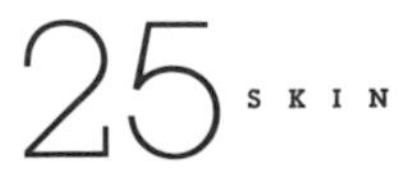

Rule of Thumb:

With sensitive skin, if you notice any change in your skin—if you've broken out or your skin is irritated or blotchy, stop using all makeup and give your skin a rest. Then add products, one by one, observing how your skin reacts to each of them.

Exfoliate regularly. Oily skin needs to be swept clean. Retina-A, developed by a dermatologist at the University of Pennsylvania School of Medicine to treat acne cases, is an excellent exfoliant for oily skin, but use it only under a physician's supervision.

Oily skin tends to break out more often than other skin types. Oil is the body's natural response of androgens—male hormones—which are secreted from the adrenal glands and the ovaries. Stress can stimulate these glands and trick them into producing more androgens. Typically, doctors treat hormonal imbalances with corticosteroids or birth control pills. They also treat adult eruptions of acne topically with benzoyl peroxide, tetracycline, or erythromycin creams; or orally with antibiotics such as tetracycline or erythromycin. Natural medicaments such as tea tree oil and cucumber or apple extracts work on mild zits. You can treat blackheads with regular deep-cleansing facials, topical benzoyl peroxide (which kills bacteria), and Retin-A.

In choosing cosmetics, look for oil-free foundations, noncomedogenic blushers (powder is preferable to creams or gels, which will just disappear into the natural oils on your face). Use oil-inhibiting matte primers designed to go on under foundation. When your face feels like a gusher has erupted, try blotting papers. Dust your face with translucent powder fluffed on with a brush, not a puff. Powder puffs get dirty, and smooshing powder into your face with them blocks pores.

Care of Sensitive Skin

This is all about risk aversion, a study in avoidance. Stay away from fragrance, fruit acids, exfoliating enzymes (no papaya masks for you), vitamins, plant extracts, preservatives, and strong soaps. Cleanse with gentle, milky, water-soluble lotions and tepid water; avoid gels that contain drying alcohol. Avoid hot water, washcloths, and scrubs. Look for products that contain natural soothers like chamomile, lavender, or jojoba. Forget about toners unless they've been formulated for sensitive skin.

Moisturizer is essential to protect sensitive skin. It must be as pure as possible, hypoallergenic, and fragrance free. Avoid products that contain a lot

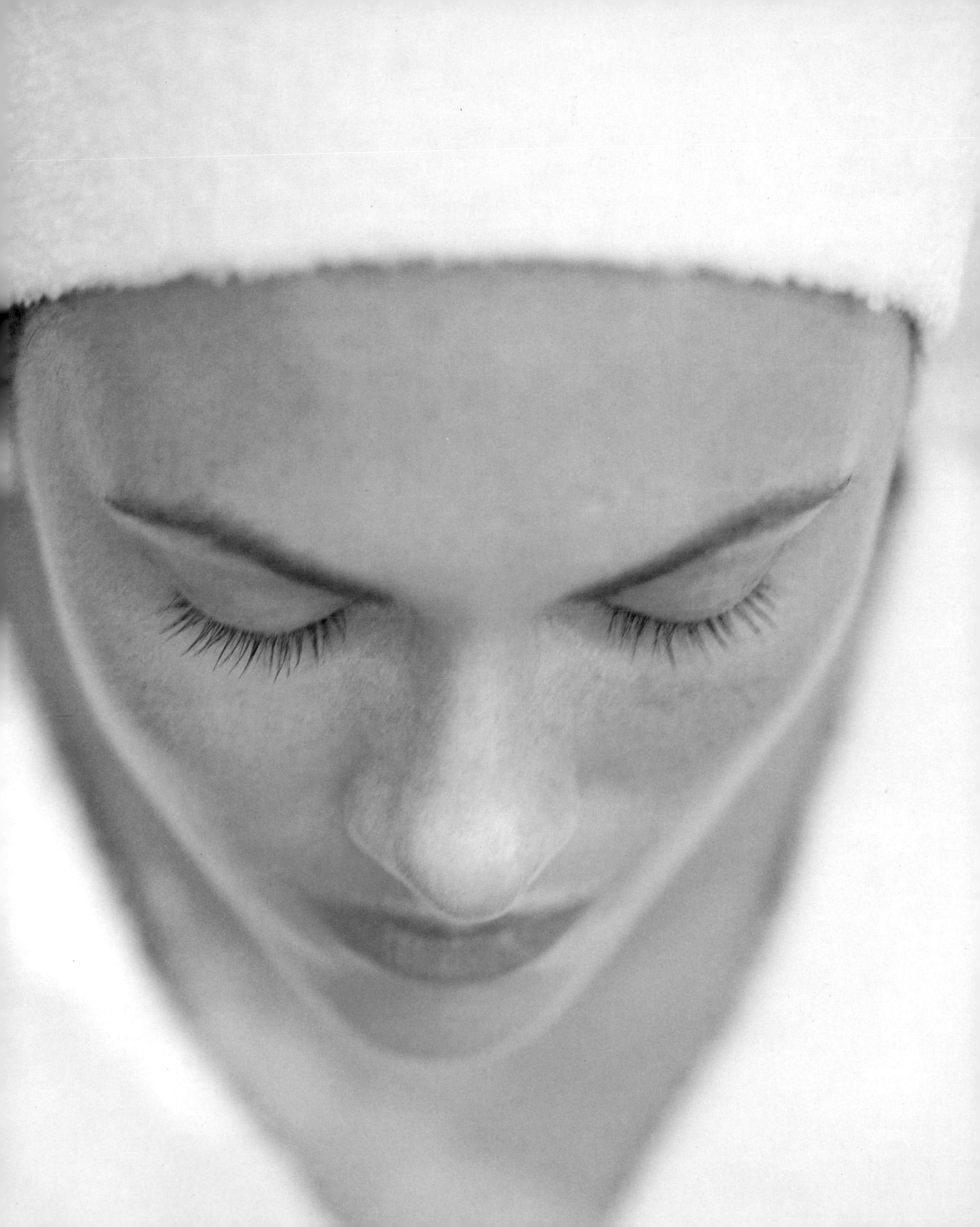

of stabilizers. Chemicals that add to the shelf life of a product wreak havoc with sensitive skin.

Many women with sensitive skin will not even attempt cosmetics, but there are some excellent oil-free, hypoallergenic foundations and fragrance-free sheer face powders available.

Care of Aging Skin

Treat your skin with gentleness and respect. Eat right. That means trading french fries for foods high in antioxidants (which attack free radicals) like green, leafy veggies; orange and yellow fruits and vegetables; and cruciferous vegetables—cabbage, kale, broccoli, and Brussels sprouts, which are also high in calcium and potassium. Drink a lot of water. Exercise regularly (long walks, stretch classes, and light weights). Get enough uninterrupted sleep. Use a gentle, nondrying cleanser. Avoid soap and alcohol-based gels. Find a water-soluble cream or lotion cleanser and use it with tepid, not hot, water. Pat your face dry with a clean, fluffy towel.

Minimal makeup looks best on aging skin. Start with a moisturizer with SPF 15 and get into the habit of using both day and night creams. Since the skin around the eyes is the thinnest on the face and the most subject to showing age (fine lines and creases), use an eye cream tapped on gently with the pad of your ring finger (supposedly the weakest of your digits). Try not to pull the skin around the eyes; this means using an eye liner pencil may be a thing of the past. Find a sheer, emollient foundation, perhaps a moisture formula. Use a light hand when applying it, because excess foundation has a way of migrating into wrinkles and fine lines. Rethink your eye makeup and stick to neutral shadows and a light whisk of mascara. Matte lipsticks are drying and highly colored ones might feather into the fine lines that develop around the mouth. Finish your makeup with a light fluff of powder applied with a soft, full brush, not a puff.

Once a week, at night before you apply night cream, use an exfoliant like an AHA, BHA, or over-the-counter retinol product. In the daytime, before you moisturize, try an antioxidant serum that contains vitamin C.

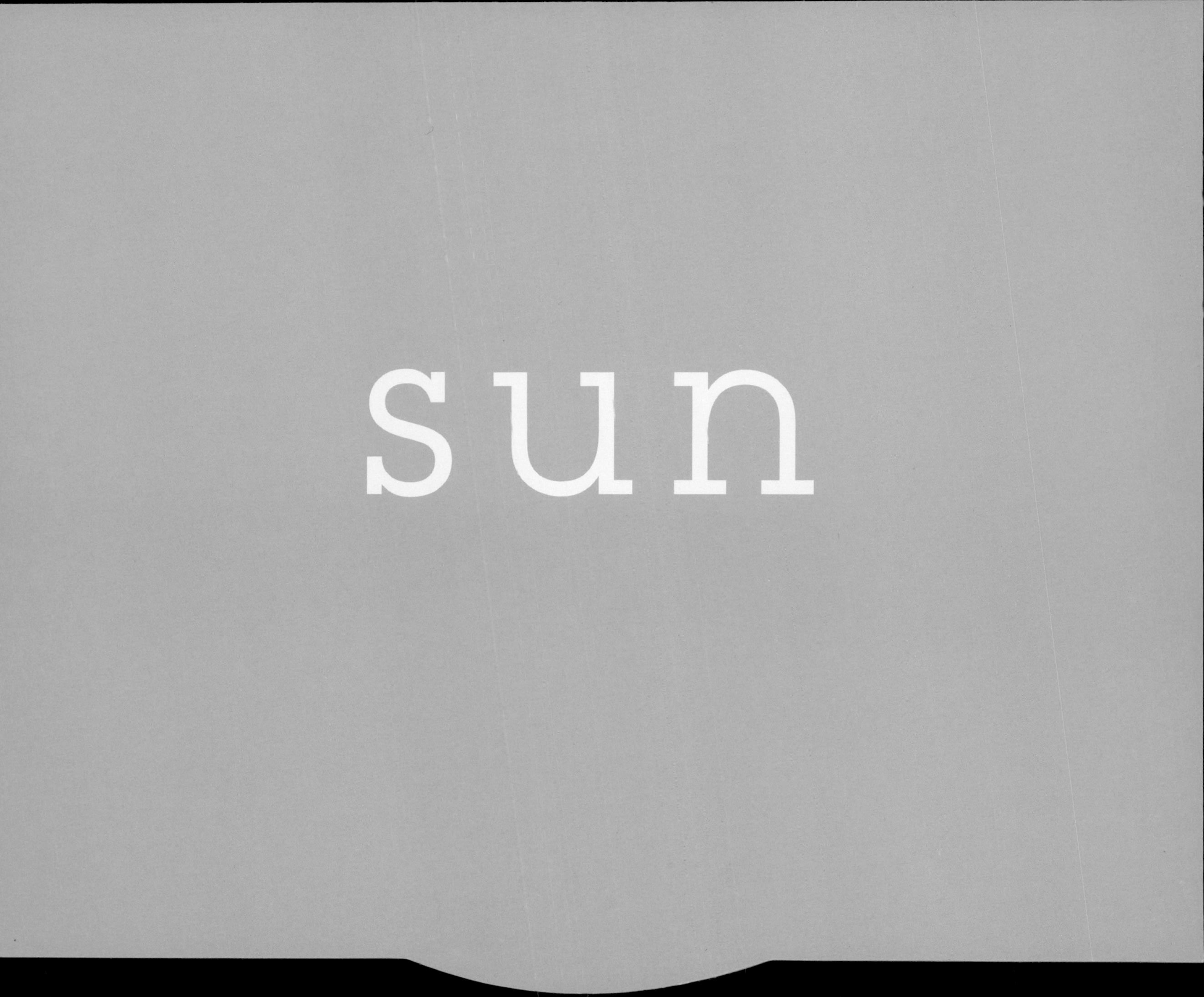
sun

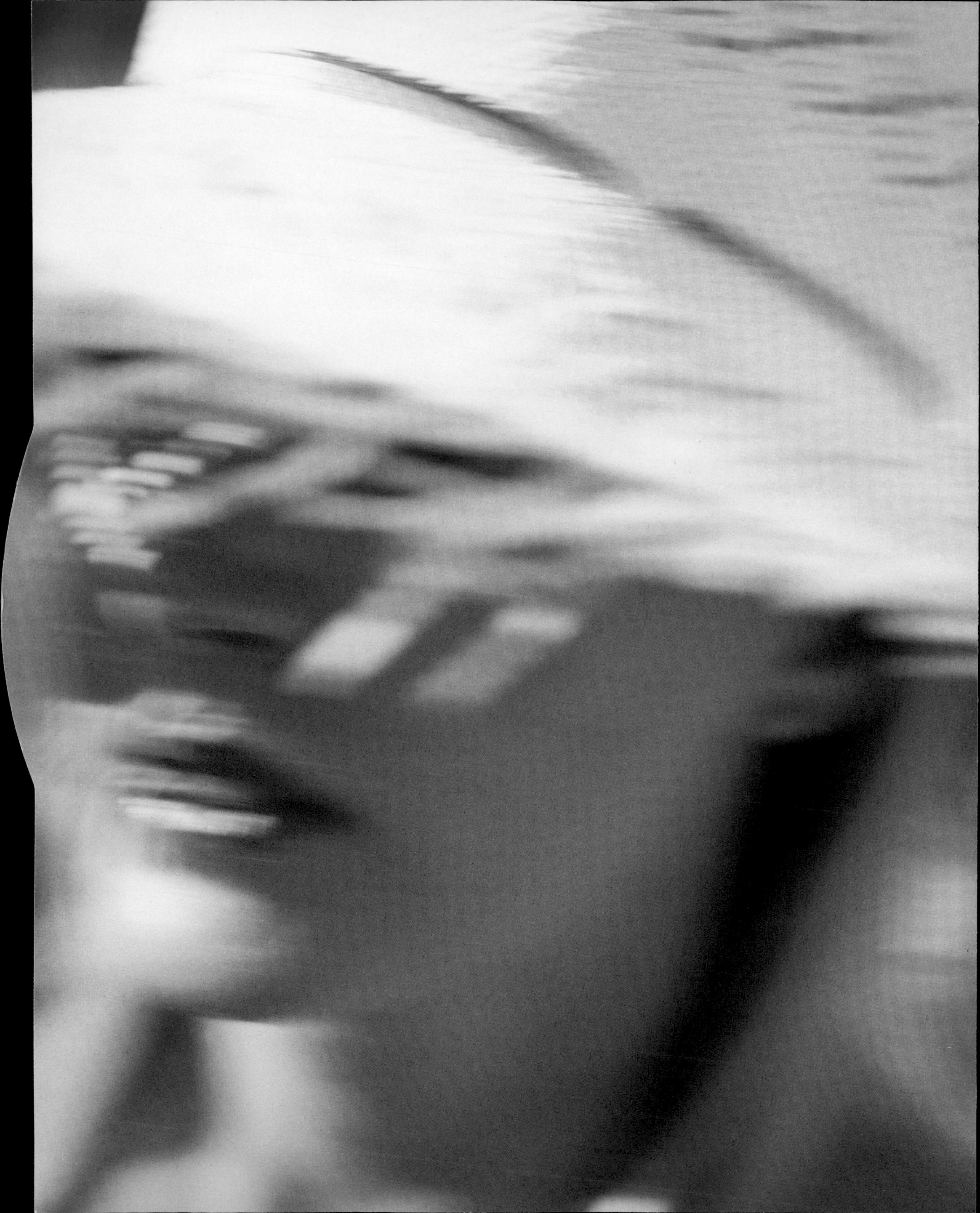

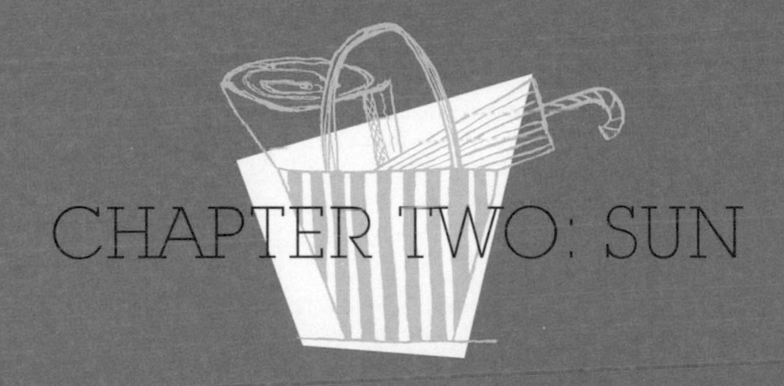

CHAPTER TWO: SUN

How can something that feels *soooo* good be so bad for you?

I'm referring to the sensation of sun on skin. Pleasant. Comforting. Warm. Sensual. Even sexy. Sunshine lifts your spirits. It adds a healthy glow to your skin. The sun's return after a long, arduous winter of rain, snow, sleet, and cold, and short, dark days restores a sense of well-being.

Medical evidence, however, shows that the sun is neither as benign nor as friendly as we'd always thought. Sun exposure is the major cause of premature skin aging. A shocking 80 percent of all skin cancers, the most easily preventable cancers, are caused by sun exposure. As we get older, the carefree days of childhood and youth spent in the swimming pool or at the beach with minimal sun protection exact their price in wrinkled, sagging, dry, and cloudy skin, and in cancers that can be lethal if undetected or untreated.

We've been brainwashed about sunshine: It makes the flowers grow. Without it, the earth would be barren and uninhabitable. The sun is the happiest of symbols, one that shows up in pop lyrics or as the iconic happy face, the bouncy, elated, chrome-yellow orb.

Given all the dermatological evidence that sun exposure is the single most damaging and aging factor for the skin, I wish I had never sat in the sun. When I was a teenager, I spent long summer days oiled up like a camshaft, turning pink, then red, then brown. My tan lines were like stripes of rank or medals of honor. My skin tanned easily; my complexion was a lovely golden brown. I looked great in coral lipstick. But did I ever equate the tender skin on my nose, which was perpetually blistered and peeling, with sun damage?

Scientists and physicians began to recognize the correlation between sunshine and skin cancer more than 25 years ago. It has taken much longer for the general population to catch on. And the price has been steep. Skin cancer rates are the highest they have ever been. The agencies that track these figures now say the chances are one in seven that you will get some form of skin cancer in your lifetime.

The sun, therefore, is nothing to mess with. The surface of our ruling star, the center of our solar system, is punctuated by violent nuclear explosions that send dangerous rays earthward through the atmosphere. Our ozone layer deflects and defuses many of these rays, but holes in the ozone caused by environmental pollutants have made even minimal sun exposure—like simply walking across a parking lot—an increasingly risky proposition.

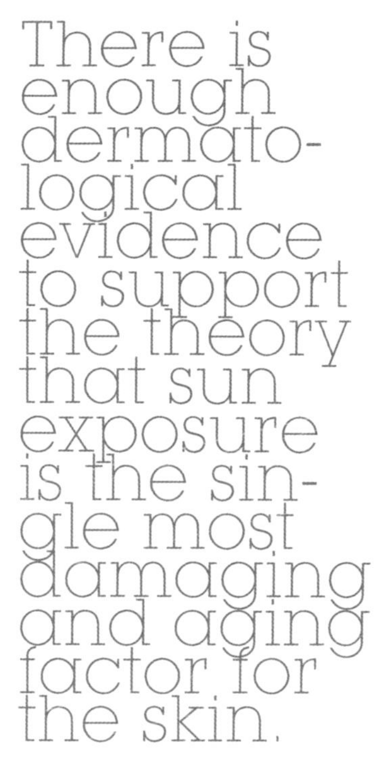
There is enough dermatological evidence to support the theory that sun exposure is the single most damaging and aging factor for the skin.

When you sit in the sun, a number of things can happen. The sun's rays raise *melanocytes*, the color-producing cells close to the surface of the skin. If you get a slight sunburn, the effects will show up immediately, probably as pinkness or redness and minor discomfort. Your skin may itch and feel tender or stretched. These are nature's ways of telling you to head for shelter. Over a longer period of time, however, the sun's more treacherous effects show up. It may take 20 years, but the result of undisciplined sun exposure is photo aging—loss of elasticity, sun spots, lines, and wrinkles—and possibly skin cancer. Look at people over 40 who have spent a lot of time in the sun gardening, playing tennis, swimming, boating, skiing, or golfing without using sunscreens religiously; their skin will appear dry and leathery. They will usually have fine lines around their eyes (which can start showing up at age 30, by the way), wrinkles, and in extreme cases, skin discolorations. Ironically, and in some cases, tragically, most of these conditions could have been prevented altogether, but they cannot be reversed without an expensive surgical process.

It is hard to change the habits of a lifetime. You love the sun, and you love to look healthy. You love how robust and even sexy a suntan makes you look and feel. Sunshine, in moderation and with the right kind of sun protection—whether a sophisticated product with a high sun-protection factor or a simple baseball cap—can enhance your sense of well-being. Humans require a modicum of vitamin D daily for good mental and physical health. But 15 minutes of limited exposure early in the morning or after 3 P.M. will supply all the delicious vitamin D you need.

Sunshine, in moderation and with the right kind of sun protection—whether a sophisticated product with a high sun protection factor or a simple baseball cap—can enhance your sense of well-being.

In this chapter, you will learn how the sun's rays can impact your skin and how to prevent both the aging effects of the sun and skin cancer. You'll also gain (I hope) a healthy respect for sunshine. You'll learn how to choose the right sun product for your skin type, what "SPF" means, and how to gauge which SPF number is right for you.

The suntan—for many years the fashion press's standard for sizzling glamour—is literally fading in importance. Sun-product advertisers now tout protection rather than intense bronzing. Advertisements in slick magazines for sun products show models many shades lighter than they once did. Finally, the consumer's eye is acclimating to the lighter shade of pale.

The advent of sunless tanners has also converted the process of tanning into a cosmetic affectation rather than an activity that puts skin in peril. You'll learn the ins and outs of faking a tan, what the labels mean, which product is right for you, and how to apply one.

In the following pages, you will improve your "Sun-Q" considerably. Since we belong to a society that thinks, "If a little is good, a lot must be better," let us err on the side of caution. Respect the sun, take the proper precautions, and your skin will thank you for it.

BRIEF HISTORY OF THE SUNTAN

In earlier centuries, paleness in European women was considered a mark of good breeding. Only peasants and slaves who worked in the fields bore the effects of the sun, earning ruddy, weathered faces and hands.

Through the centuries, nothing much changed. Women were controlled by the men in their lives and revered for their delicate, ghostly pallor. When they did use cosmetics—as women were wont to do from the time of Cleopatra to the prissy Victorians—they lightened their complexions even more by coating their faces with a toxic mixture called ceruse, which contained white lead.

By the Victorian era, makeup had become frowned upon as sexually subversive and frivolous. The proper Victorians hid their faces under parasols, covered their décolletage with high collars or bits of lace, and protected their hands in leather or cotton gloves. When they went bathing at the shore, they sat under massive beach umbrellas and wore woolen bathing costumes with mobcaps over their curls. Thus protected from impropriety, Victorian women remained sun-proofed and pale.

After the turn of the century and World War I, women entered the workforce and began liberating themselves. In America, they won the right to vote. In the 1920s, they threw off their corsets, tied down their breasts, shortened their skirts, bobbed their hair, smoked cigarettes, drank martinis, and raised some flapper hell. Out of the Roaring Twenties came the ultimate French flapper, the upstart of haute couture—Coco Chanel. Coco fled to the sun one particularly bad winter in Paris, and when she returned from vacationing with such society darlings as the Duke and Duchess of Windsor on the Côte d'Azur on the French Riviera, her face and body had tanned to a fetching bronze. Since Mlle. Chanel was the style setter of the time, she changed the course of dermatological history for at least 50 years. And not all for the best.

The suntan became the status symbol of the idle rich. An out-of-season tan meant that you had the funds, the social rank, and the leisure time to vacation in tropical climes while the work-a-day world was busy slaving away and slogging through the sleet and slush. In the late 1930s, bathing costumes became more abbreviated bathing suits, showing more skin. Suntan lotions hit the market in the mid-1940s, after World War II. But their focus was on maximum exposure, not protection. Fashion aided and abetted the suntan when, in the mid-1950s, the bikini appeared. Often three daring triangles of fabric held on by the narrowest of straps, the bikini flirted with seminudity, affording just enough material to keep the wearer from getting kicked off the beach.

Starting in the mid-1970s, however, physicians began noting a precipitous rise in the occurrence of skin cancers, particularly malignant melanoma. They made the correlation between sun exposure and skin cancer. Dermatologists also noted that although the sun gave women an attractive, healthy glow, it also aged their skin faster. The small lines around the mouth

When Coco Chanel came back from the French Riviera with a tan in the 1920s, she changed the course of dermatological history for at least 50 years.

How many middle-aged women still think they look better, healthier, sexier with a suntan?

and eyes that normally appear after age 30 became serious wrinkles with regular sun exposure. As the supportive tissue of the skin lost its bounce, faces sagged and bagged. By age 40, women's girlish pink complexions started exhibiting unattractive discoloration and freckles, and their hands and chests appeared tattooed with uneven brown spots.

In the late 1970s, the scientific community reported on a serious problem in the ozone layer, the only protection between earth and the powerfully lethal rays of the sun. The thinning of the ozone layer has been linked to pollution and waste, such as gases from aerosol spray cans, industrial pollutants, solvents, plastic, and styrofoam. Now the sun could do far more damage in less time.

Fashion had dictated the rise of the suntan. And fashion magazines have finally taken up the banner of sun protection and have changed women's perceptions of what is attractive. The latest message—sent by articles and advertisements featuring lighter-skinned models—is that pallor is pretty. Not to mention safe. It's difficult, however, to give up the habits of a lifetime. How many middle-aged women still think they look better, healthier, sexier with a suntan?

To accommodate changing health factors concerning the sun, cosmetic companies have come up with effective no-sun tanners—not the awful orange veggie dyes of the 1960s, but products that are easy to apply and approximate an actual tan without the sun's harmful effects.

Self-tanning will never take the place of a real suntan. But the rules about sitting in the sun have also changed. Sunscreens and physical sunblocks allow for sensible, moderate sun exposure. That Mexican or Hawaiian vacation can still be an enjoyable option if you know the rules. Today's sun-protection products are far superior to those of 10 years ago.

You'll not see women returning to parasols, white gloves, and woolen bathing costumes in the near future, but you will see protective clothing, caps and hats, timed sun exposure, and tote bags stuffed with sun creams, gels, oils, lotions, and aprés-sun soothers to make tanning a lot less hazardous to their health.

Ultraviolet Light

Telescopic photographs of the sun show rays, hundreds of miles long, shooting off its surface. They emit a spectrum of radiant energy measured in different wavelengths, some of which are in the ultraviolet spectrum. These are invisible and harmful to humans.

Ultraviolet rays exist in three measurable lengths and intensities: ultraviolet A (UVA), ultraviolet B (UVB), and ultraviolet C (UVC). UVCs are the shortest and most lethal UV rays. Fortunately, the ozone layer prevents them from hitting the earth's surface. It is with UVAs and UVBs that we should be concerned.

UVBs cause sunburn and are considered the principal contributors to basal and squamous-cell carcinoma as well as the major factors in the development of malignant melanomas, cataracts, and immune-system damage. In the mnemonic of sun care: *UVB = burning.*

UVAs are an entirely different story, and until the early 1980s were considered the "safe" sun ray. Medical practice has since proven otherwise. Longer than the UVBs, UVAs are more insidious. They reach right through auto and window glass, speed through 9 feet of water, and penetrate cloud layers; so that even on gray, misty, or stormy days, your skin gets sun exposure. UVAs are the rays inherent in ostensibly safe indoor tanning beds and sunlamps which have proven not to be so safe after all. The effects of UVA exposure may not show up for 20 years, but much of the damage is irreversible without a physician's help. UVAs were once considered merely aging factors, but recently they've also been implicated in skin cancers, including melanoma. In the mnemonic of sun care: *UVA = aging.*

Consider the alarming facts about sun exposure to be a heads up to educate yourself about sun, to respect its power, and to act accordingly. When you expose your skin to sun, UVBs hit you first and are absorbed by the epidermis, generating free radicals, which destroy cells or cause cell mutation. Besides turning your skin shrimp pink or an ouchy lobster red, UVBs will work their dastardly deeds inside the body.

Sounding the Alarm about Sun Exposure

Sunshine has a deleterious effect on human skin. Here are some alarming facts to keep in mind:

- **Up to 80 percent of the visible signs of aging on the face can be traced directly to the sun.**
- **Skin cancer is the fastest-growing cancer in the United States.**
- **More than a million new cases of skin cancer are diagnosed each year.**
- **Dermatologists estimate that if 10 percent of Americans now using some kind of SPF sun product were to stop, there would be an additional million cases of skin cancer each year.**

How Sun Protection Factor (SPF) Works

On the market are broad-spectrum sun protection products that screen and block both UVB and UVA rays. The higher the number, the more effective the product. On a sunscreen package, the SPF tells you how much longer you can stay in the sun without burning. SPF 15 allows you to remain in the sun 15 times longer than if you didn't have sunscreen on. If you burn in 10 minutes, with SPF 15, you can theoretically stay in the sun 150 minutes. With SPF 30, your time in the sun can increase, but so do the ray-stopping properties of the protection, which means less color. Products with SPF 45, in fact, render almost no sun exposure (or color) to the skin, as they physically block all of the sun's rays.

UVAs penetrate deeply into the body—40 times deeper than UVB rays, wresting life-supporting oxygen molecules apart to create free radicals. Like time bombs, free radicals look for a place to explode, causing collagen collapse, skin discoloration, and precancerous conditions. UVAs are also the culprits behind photo aging.

While the news on profligate sun exposure is not good, there is, as cosmetic companies are wont to say, hope in a jar. And in a tube, in a spray applicator, or in a bottle. That hope is called sunblock.

SUN PROTECTION

Sunscreens were originally invented in the 1940s when the whole idea was to *promote* a tan, not avoid it. The choices then were cream, oil, or lotion. Today, the roster of products is myriad and confusing. There are both sunscreens and sunblocks, which come in gels, lotions, creams, sticks, mousses, and sprays. They include oil-free, hypoallergenic, and active sports formulas. There are products for babies and children as well as separate formulas for faces and other specific parts of the body (noses and part lines, for instance). How do you choose the right one for you?

Any sun protection product with an SPF 2 or higher is considered a sunscreen; the active ingredient is a chemical. Any product with SPF 12 or higher will contain a physical sunblock. Sunscreen chemicals are designed to combine with your skin chemistry to mitigate the harsh rays of the sun. They protect the skin from UVB rays but provide incomplete protection against UVAs. Read your labels. Sunscreens contain any or a combination of the following: octyl methoxycinnamate (OMC), octocrylene salicylate (OCS), PABA (para-aminobenzoic acid), octyl dimethyl PABA (Padimate), oxybenzone (bezophenone-3), and avobenzone (Parsol 1789). Because these chemical sun inhibitors are designed to be absorbed by the epidermis and are metabolized in the body, they invariably cause allergic reactions—rashes and redness and maybe some pimples. (If you get any kind of physical reaction from a cosmetic product, stop using it immediately!)

Sunblocks, on the other hand, sit on the surface of the skin and physically block both UVB and some UVA rays. Call them your skin's crossing guards. There are two of them: zinc oxide (readily recognizable as the viscous white goop that lifeguards wear on their noses) and titanium dioxide.

Titanium dixoide, the most common sunblock, completely protects skin from UVB radiation and offers limited UVA protection—slowing down or stopping everything but the longest, most lethal rays of the UVA spectrum. Using zinc oxide, however, is like sitting on the beach fully clothed, so complete is its protection. It is also aesthetically unpleasant—white, thick, and obvious on the skin. A number of companies now use a form of zinc oxide in which the molecule has been rendered small enough to appear invisible on the skin (look for the product Z-Cote in the list of ingredients).

Starting in the mid-1970s, physicians began noting a precipitous rise in the occurrence of skin cancers.

Chemical Sunscreen Ingredients

- **Octyl methoxycinnamate (OMC).** The most common chemical sunscreen in the world. Blocks UVBs only.
- **Octocrylene.** Blocks UVBs only.
- **Octocrylene salicylate (OCS).** Used with other ingredients to increase SPF. A very weak UVB block if used alone.
- **PABA (para-aminobenzoic acid).** Once thought to be the most effective of the chemical blocks, but it caused allergic reactions and rashes and was taken off the market. PABA blocked only UVB rays.
- **Octyl dimethyl PABA (Padimate-O).** Developed as an alternative to PABA. Blocks only UVB rays.
- **Oxybenzone (benzophenone-3).** Designed to block UVA rays, but it causes allergic reactions.
- **Avobenzone (Parsol 1789).** Blocks partial UVA rays; not as effective by itself, it is often combined in products with benzophenone-3. Also causes some allergic reactions.

Physical Sunscreen Ingredients

- **Titanium dioxide.** At higher SPF numbers, this chemical can turn white or bluish on the skin. Provides UVB protection and partial UVA protection.
- **Zinc oxide.** A nearly total sunblock providing complete protection against both UVB and UVA rays. White and pasty, it is aesthetically unpleasant to use.
- **Z-Cote.** A patented form of zinc oxide with smaller molecules, which make it transparent on the skin. Also an effective UVA/UVB block.

SKIN TYPING FOR THE RIGHT PROTECTION

When suntan creams first came out with sun protection factors, the highest number available was 15, and it was designed to screen out only the burning rays of the sun. SPF 15 blocked 93 percent of all UVBs and was, initially, the most effective way to lessen the strength of the burning rays. Cosmetic companies were in the habit of putting higher SPF numbers on their sunscreens, depending upon the amount of chemicals in the formula; but by and large, the highest protection afforded for all of them was SPF 15.

These days, higher SPF numbers actually mean something. High SPF numbers—products with values over SPF 15 to as much as SPF 45—measure the sunblocking powers of the product.

How high is *your* SPF? How high *should* it be? What kind of protection do you really need? The first step is to determine your skin type and then buy a product that will give you optimum protection. Modern sunscreens come with higher and more accurate SPF numbers that reflect the protection within. If you are fair-skinned and burn easily, using products with SPF 30 to SPF 45 is imperative.

Skin Types*

Type I	Always burns, never tans
Type II	Burns easily, tans minimally
Type III	Burns moderately, tans gradually to light brown
Type IV	Rarely burns, tans profusely to dark brown
Type V	Never burns, deeply pigmented

* *According to the American Academy of Dermatology and the Food and Drug Administration*

If your skin type falls between types I and II, you probably have very fair, thin skin that is on the dry side, blue eyes, and lighter hair. In the sun, you freckle and burn quickly. You are also at a much higher risk for skin cancer. With fair skin your sun protection should be SPF 30 or higher, depending upon whether you want to get some color. There are certain types of sun products that go to SPF 45 and higher, which will prevent any kind of skin coloring. With skin types III and higher, your SPF number can be lower. If you live or work in the mountains, where the atmosphere is thinner, the sun is much stronger. Regardless of your skin type, choose a higher number sun product.

Here are a few more things to remember: These products are designed to be used generously and often. When you are outside, whether you are simply sunning or exerting yourself playing tennis, working in the garden, or swimming, you must reapply your sunscreen often, because you're rinsing, swimming, toweling, or sweating it off. Use a lot and coat your exposed parts thoroughly. Other factors to consider when choosing a sun-protection product could include whether it is waterproof, water resistant, sweatproof, hypoallergenic, or noncomedogenic.

When you apply sun protection, be generous. It can't work if you don't use it right. Stroke, spray, or foam it on (whichever form you prefer) over clean skin, and try not to rub it in too much. Sunscreens should be allowed to dry for about 20 minutes *before* you get any sun exposure. If you're swimming or sweating, be sure to reapply, generously and often. Even if you're not exercising, it's wise to apply more sun product every hour or so. If you are extravagant about any part of your sun rituals, let it be the amount of sun protection you use.

Products for Different Activities and Skin Sensitivities*

- **Waterproof, water resistant.** You can expect up to 80 minutes of protection from a waterproof sunscreen, 40 minutes from a water-resistant one. Use these while swimming, boating, waterskiing, or fishing. Reapply often.
- **Sweatproof.** These products bond on contact with skin; they are nongreasy and slip proof. If you use the product on your face, it shouldn't run into your eyes and sting (if it does, quit using it). Sweatproof products are ideal for tennis, golf, jogging, and gardening, any time when you might perspire heavily.
- **Hypoallergenic.** These products are easy on the skin and are designed for people with sensitive skin or for children.
- **Noncomedogenic.** This word on the label usually means that there are cosmetic-grade ingredients in the product. They are found in products designed for use on the face, not the body. Usually, you will not get whiteheads, blackheads, bumps, or clogged pores from these products. They are especially good for oily and breakout-prone skin.

*From the Coppertone Solar Research Center

Rule of Thumb:

Reapply sunscreens and sunblocks at least once an hour regardless of your physical activity. And be sure to use liberal amounts.

Like milk and eggs, sunscreens have a limited shelf life. The expiration date is printed on the bottle. Keep your sunscreen out of the sun and store it in a cool, dry place. Don't keep half-used bottles lying around at the end of the sun season in a golf bag or at the bottom of your beach carryall. Toss them out and buy new ones at the beginning of the next season or right before you take a vacation in the sun.

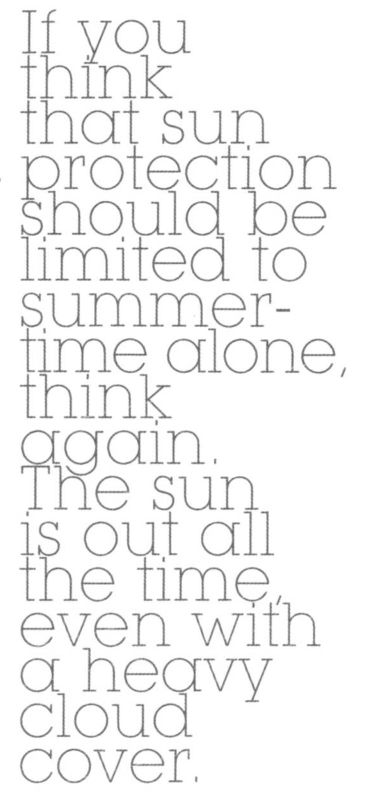
If you think that sun protection should be limited to summer-time alone, think again. The sun is out all the time, even with a heavy cloud cover.

If you think that sun protection should be limited to summertime alone, think again. The sun is out all the time, even with a heavy cloud cover. Dermatologists repeat the mantra: *Sunscreen. Don't leave home without it.* Wisely, cosmetic companies have picked up the beat and are putting SPFs in their moisturizers, foundations, and even lipsticks. The minimum protection is probably an SPF 8. Don't buy anything less. You might find, however, that products with SPF in them may be comedogenic—that is, they could block your pores, causing breakouts, whiteheads, and blackheads. If that happens, put a separate sunscreen product over your moisturizer instead of buying an all-in-one product. Just like brushing your teeth, putting on sunscreen should be an automatic part of your daily routine.

Of additional importance are the weave and color of the clothes you wear, the brim-circumference on your hat, and your sunglasses. Clothes should be lightweight but of a tight weave—they should cast a shadow when you hold them up to the light. Baseball caps are great if you have long hair that covers the back of your neck and ears; otherwise, trade them in for broad-brimmed, tightly woven straw hats.

As for sunglasses, go for protection, not for style. Those trendy John Lennon specs may be cool for the clubs, but as sunblockers, they are totally inappropriate. Make sure that the lenses cover your eyes from the brow to about half an inch below the eye. The skin around your eyes is the thinnest and most delicate. It is also the area on your face that shows damage first. A wraparound frame with wide temple bars will protect your eyes and the skin around them. Look for UV-rated lenses that are optically ground (much easier to see through and better for your eyes). Save yellow lenses for skiing; opt for gray, dark green, brown, or black tints.

Your Sun-Q Quick Checklist for Sun Safety*

① Avoid the sun between 10 a.m. and 3 p.m. (11 a.m. and 4 p.m. daylight saving time).

② Apply a broad-spectrum sunscreen or a sunblock with an SPF of at least 15 that shields both UVA and UVB rays.

③ Reapply sunblock generously when you swim, sweat, or towel off; at least every hour, even on overcast days.

④ Wear protective clothing: tight-weave, long-sleeved shirts and pants.

⑤ Wear a hat with a large brim that protects the back of your neck as well as your face and ears.

⑥ Wear sunglasses with lenses that block out 100 percent of UV rays with frames that wrap around your face.

⑦ Reflective surfaces can refract up to 85 percent of the sun's rays, so coat up with SPF 15 if you're going to be near water, concrete, sand, or snow (or even the shiny tabletop of your favorite sidewalk café).

⑧ Avoid using sunscreen on infants under six months old; keep them out of the sun entirely. Even if you're walking with them in a stroller, protect them with long sleeves, pants, and a floppy-brimmed hat.

⑨ Make sure teenagers understand the long-term damage that unprotected sun exposure can cause. Teach them early and well and get them into the habit of using sun protection and common sense.

*Courtesy of the *American Academy of Dermatology*

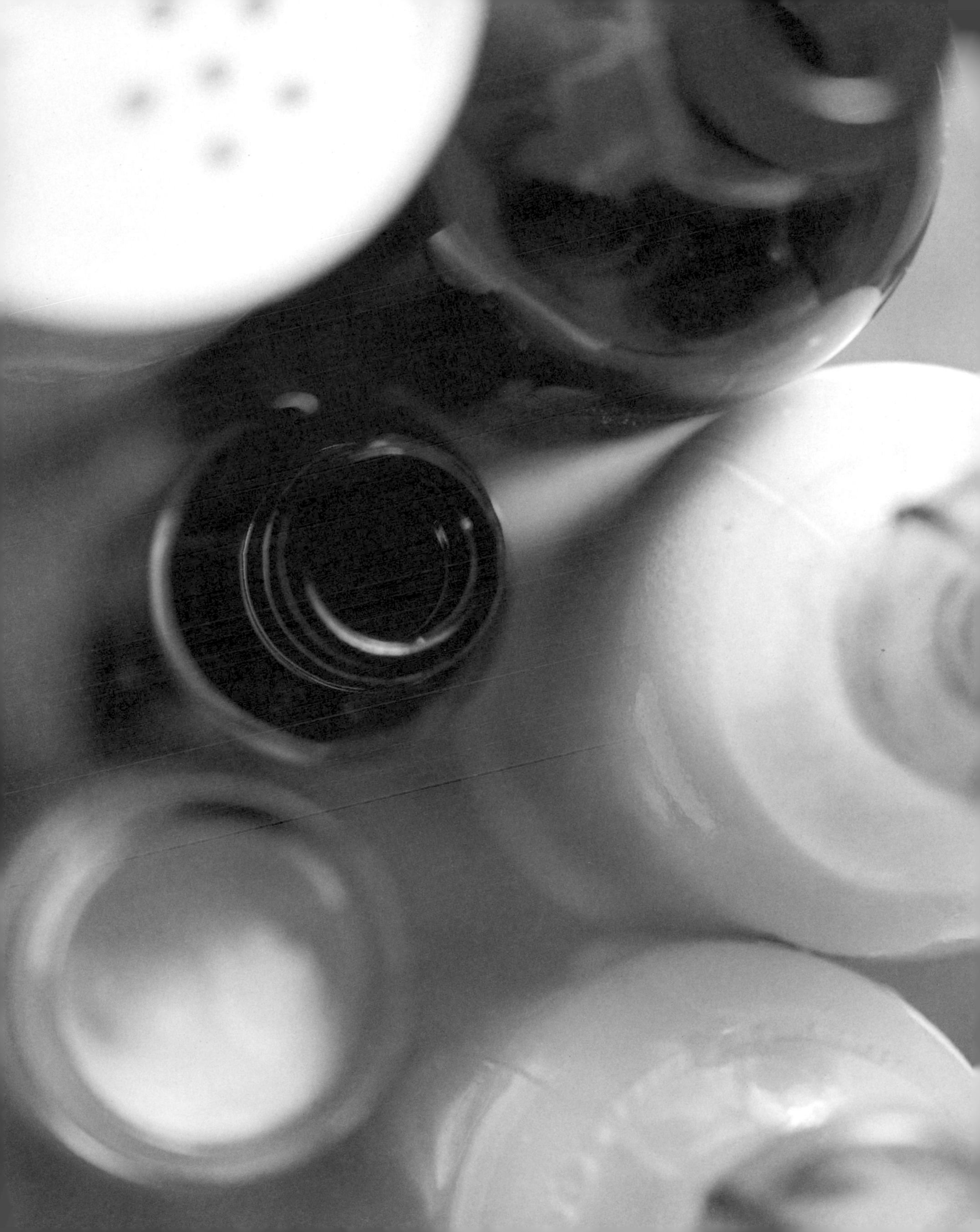

FAKING IT: TANNING WITHOUT THE SUN

No-sun tanner is probably the best invention since sliced bread, especially the ones on the market today. They are easy to use and require very little upkeep; some even smell good. Most important, they give the appearance of a great suntan but keep you away from the harmful rays of the sun.

When they first came out, they were pretty primitive cosmetics. They smelled wretched (like old nicotine crossed with stale vegetables), and they turned you some unbelievable shade of orange. Now, no-sun tanners are high-tech and refined. Good-bye, orange; hello, gorgeous.

The primary active ingredient in sunless-tanning products, called DHA, is a derivative of sugarcane or sugar beets that oxidizes with the top layer of skin by reacting with the amino proteins. It is not a vegetable dye. While DHA bonds with the top few layers of the skin to give it a tan appearance, it does not penetrate the skin at all. Research carried on for years at huge cosmetic companies indicates that these products are harmless and have no cancer-causing potential.

One word of warning, however: *No-sun tanners provide absolutely zero sun protection.* Since they are strictly a cosmetic, they do not alter the structure or function of the skin, nor do they raise the melanin production in your skin. And no, they are not an automatic shield against sunlight. So if you've used a tanner and want to go out in the sun, you still have to use sun protection. The biggest downside to using a no-sun tanner is the false sense of security that some users are lulled into: Many believe that the darker your skin gets, the more you're protected. But it simply does not work that way. Another downside is that excessive sweat will make these fakers streak and run on the skin.

No-sun tanners fade as your body sheds dead skin cells. Every time you bathe or shower, or use a loofah or even a towel, your tan fades, which means that every two to three days, you need to reapply the tanner to refresh your tan.

There are a variety of no-sun tanners on the market now—formulas for light, medium, or dark tans, as well as for sensitive skin. They are available in many forms: spray-on oil, foam, mousse, lotion, gel, and cream. Try out a no-sun tanner in the smallest size available. Otherwise, you could end up with a bag filled with barely used products that you didn't like.

Test the tanner first by applying it on a limited area below your jawline or on your inner arm. If you're happy with the results, continue your application. If you're not, you'll have to try another brand. This is a highly experimental procedure. Be patient. Buy the products whose texture and odor you like and that turn you the desired shade of bronze. If you are inexperienced with no-sun tanning, some products are easier to control than others. Start out with a cream or a gel and then graduate to the more-difficult-to-control mousses, oils, or lotions. Foam mousse dries faster, but unless you get it on evenly, it can streak.

Self-tanning requires a bit of planning and specific steps during application for best results. You can't just slop the stuff on and expect to have the perfect tan. Also, you shouldn't try to use it right after you've shaved your legs, primarily to keep down the irritation level on freshly shaved skin, but also because shaving opens the pores, and the DHA will hide in them and give your tan a dotted appearance.

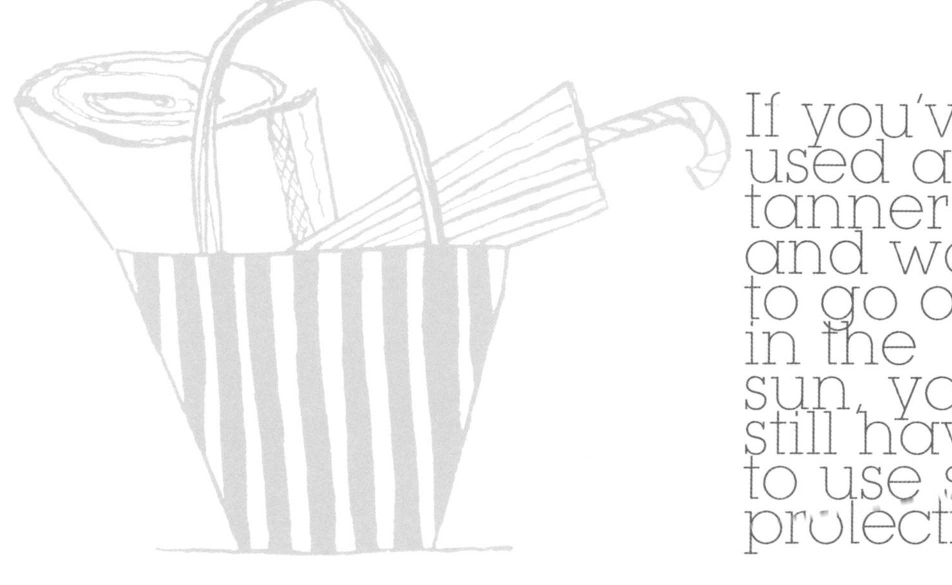

If you've used a tanner and want to go out in the sun, you still have to use sun protection.

How to use no-sun tanners effectively

1. Prepare your skin "canvas"—exfoliate: To get your skin primed and receptive for the glories of a deep, satisfying, and totally safe tanning experience, you must first exfoliate the skin to get rid of the dead cells, which could affect the color of the tan. Use a loofah or a textured scrubber (a sponge will work) and maybe a nail brush and some gentle exfoliating gel or body scrub. Before you turn on the water, climb into the shower and work the scrub around your body, concentrating on areas where your skin is the thickest—elbows, ankles, knees, wrists, and backs of heels. If you don't get these places fairly smooth, the tanner will congregate in creases and look darker there than on the rest of your body. Rinse off and towel dry.

2. Prepare your chair (or bed): Spread a large terry bath towel on a chair or on your bed; prop your pillows up against the wall and cover them with a towel as well. You're going to want to protect the space where you'll rest for half an hour sans clothing after you finish your application.

3. Protect hair and palms: Pin your hair away from your face and rub a little petroleum jelly or hair conditioner around your hairline. Use surgical or kitchen gloves to apply your tanner, removing them only when you do your hands (the last step). If you don't use gloves, wash your hands carefully, or you'll wind up with orange palms.

4. Work upward from your feet: Use copious amounts of tanner and apply it in long, even strokes; then stroke the tanner cross-ways to ensure even distribution.

⑤ Use moisturizer on the places with the thickest skin before applying tanner: This means elbows, ankles, knees, feet, and wrists, where extra tanner can cake and darken in creases.

⑥ Use tanner all over your body: If you want a bikini line, you might want to wear your bathing suit while you're doing this; otherwise, apply the tanner to your entire body. After you've done your arms, chest, and upper back, you'll find that you have "the sweetheart spot" in the center of your back—the place you can't reach without help. One way to solve the problem is to have your significant other, your mom, sister, brother, or a friend help you. Sometimes, it's fun to get together with a few friends for a spa night where you can help each other apply no-sun tanner.

⑦ Use a specially formulated tanner for your face: Do not use body tanners. They are stronger and may contain chemicals that will occlude your pores. There are many tanning products designed specifically for the tender skin of your face.

⑧ Do your hands last: Use a cosmetic sponge to stroke the tanner on your hands evenly. You can also buy an inexpensive soft paint brush to finish the job. Because you wash and dry your hands many times a day, the tanner tends to exfoliate from them quickly. You will probably have to touch up your hands more often than your body.

No-sun products take three or four hours to work. If the color isn't dark enough, plan to reapply the next day. Again, be generous and apply large amounts of tanner to clean skin. You do not have to repeat the exfoliation process for your second or even third application.

Your color will last, conservatively, four to five days. If you use a shower brush, sponge, or washcloth when you bathe, you'll notice that the color will begin to naturally slough off with your dead skin cells a bit sooner.

There are beauty salons that will apply the tanner for you. They will begin with a body scrub to exfoliate your skin and get it ready to accept the color. Then they'll slather you with tanner and allow you to dry on a towel-covered mat so the color will not rub off on your clothes. Plan to stay for at least two hours for the most effective treatment.

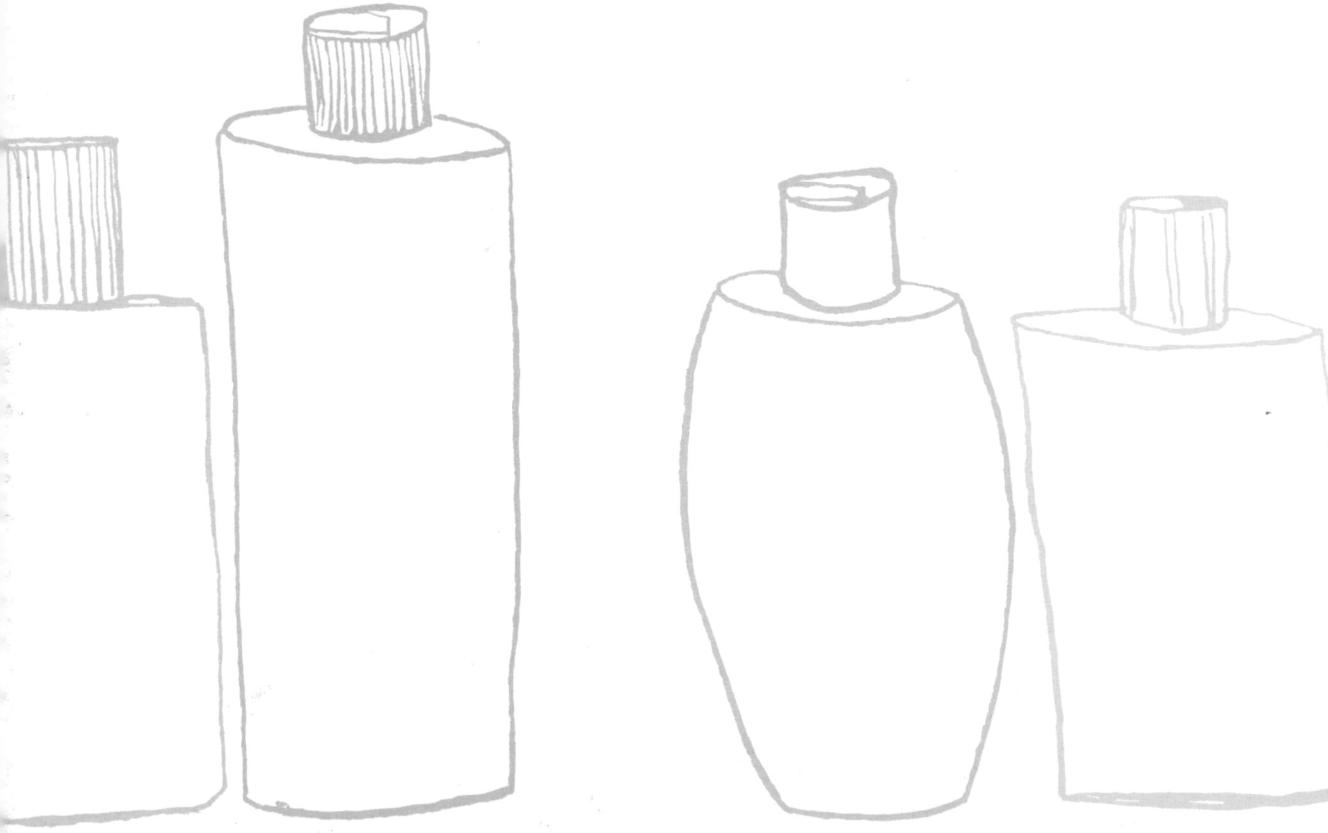

makeup

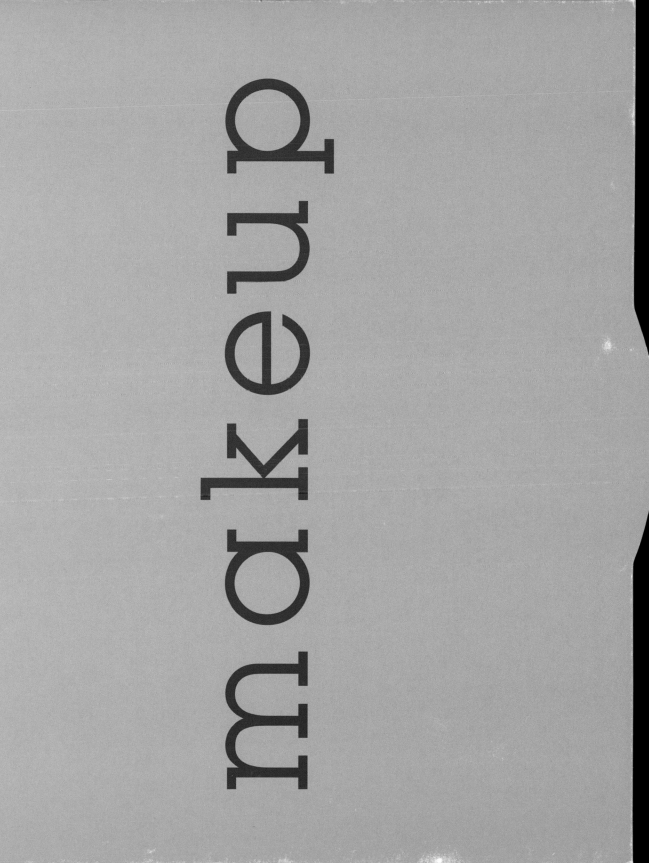

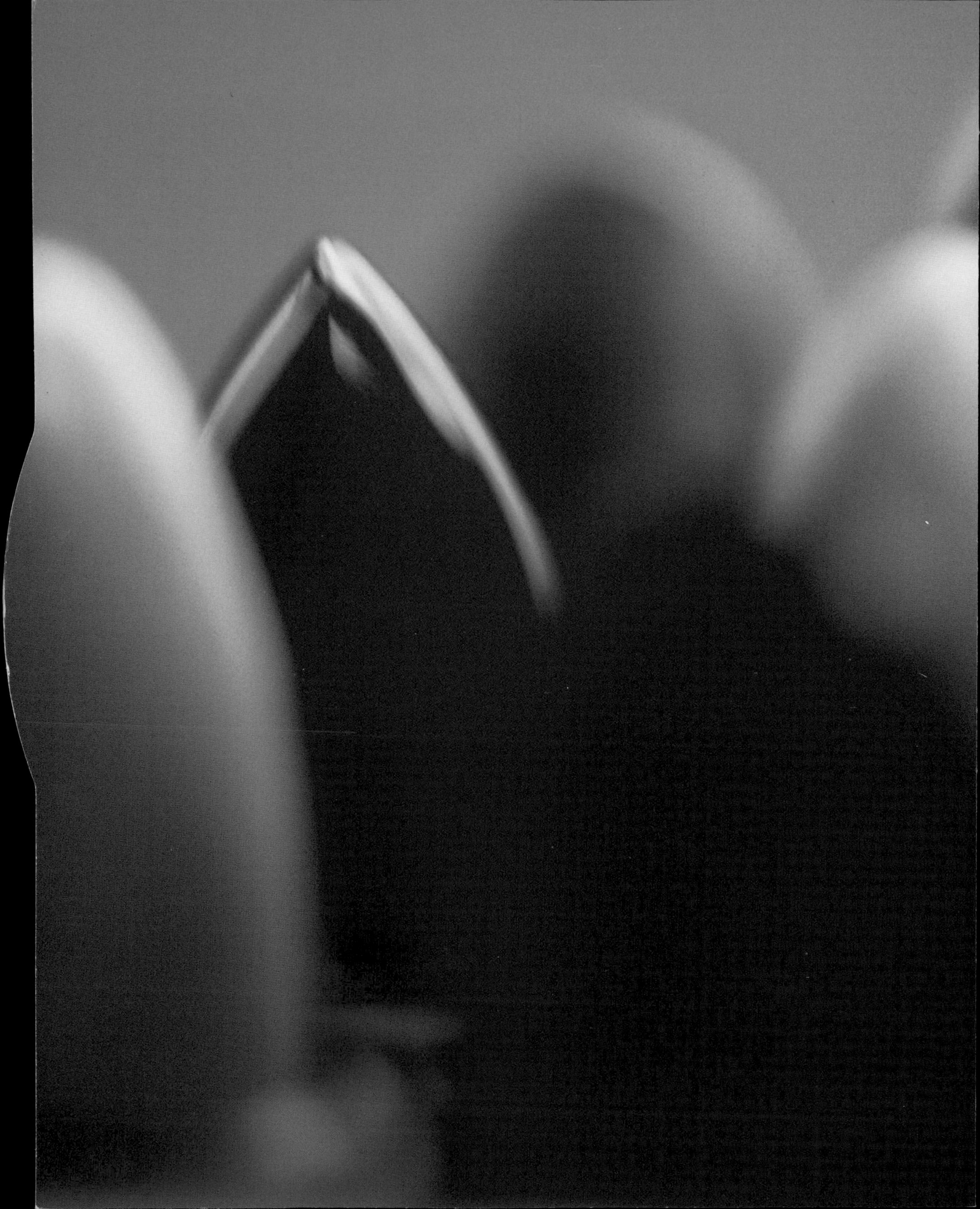

CHAPTER THREE: MAKEUP

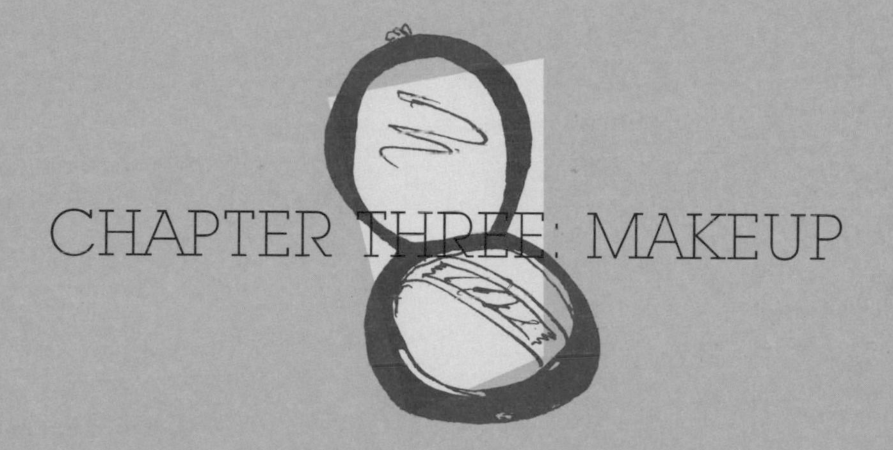

My first memory of paint and powder is of watching my mother apply cosmetics. She said she was "putting on her face," and the transition from "Mama" in her shapeless nightgown to a polished, elegant woman in perfume and high heels was always quite extraordinary.

Each morning, wrapped in a towel, she would sit in the bathroom at a mirrored vanity that my father had built for her. Fresh from the shower, her skin glowed a healthy pink. Clouds of steam scented with Estée Lauder Youth Dew bath oil swirled around her like an aura. She spent very little time in contemplation of her face, but set to work with a detached determination. If she spent more than 10 minutes doing her makeup, I would be surprised.

She never dillydallied, and each day she used the same order of application: moisturizer (Jacqueline Cochran Flowing Velvet), foundation (Estée Lauder), mascara (Maybelline), blusher (an Estée Lauder shade of pinky-rose—she kept the same one for years and years), and lipstick (Estée Lauder Persian Melon). I've often wanted to write Mrs. Lauder and thank her for making my mother beautiful.

Mama introduced me to the joys of moisturizer when I was 14 by giving me samples of Estée Lauder's yellow Youth Dew cream and then buying me my own bottles of Flowing Velvet. Considering today's lightweight moisturizers that are geared to youthful skin, these products were overkill in a bottle for a barely postpubescent teen. They may have been heavy on the oil and fragrance and much too rich for my fairly unblemished teenaged skin, but the lesson stuck. Protection and moisture were of utmost importance.

Mama was European and, like her contemporaries, was taught from babyhood to stay out of the sun and respect her skin. My Belgrade-born friend Denise Minnelli Hale, has flawless, white skin. She has not a blemish, not an age spot, not a wrinkle. She gardens and adores her roses, but in the midst of a blindingly sunny day, she's covered head to foot, hands included. Once, when Denise was a new arrival in Hollywood freshly married to a major film director, actress Eva Gabor took her aside and gave her some important advice: "Cover your hands, dah-ling. The California sun is too strong." Today, Denise laughs about how she never learned to swim, and in all of her years as a famous Hollywood hostess, never even owned a house with a pool.

My mother's prejudices about makeup were inevitably passed on to me. She was a lady and she expected me to be one too. She had prohibitions against my looking cheap and fast. While I was growing up in the Fabulous Fifties, Charles Revson was promoting one gorgeous red lipstick after another: Love That Red, Fire and Ice, Cherries in the Snow. Mama forbade me from using any of them. Instead, she would hand me her tube of Persian Melon, the most polite liptick I've ever used—a pink-heavy, slightly frosted coral—which was girlish and virginal in the extreme. Red lipsticks? They were for the girls who "put out"—sexually adventurous females of ill repute whose mothers probably weren't watching what they were doing. (I wonder how my mother would have reacted to today's teen fashions: blue hair and pierced navels.)

The great cosmetic companies of the 1950s—Revlon, Helena Rubinstein, Gala, Tangée, Charles of the Ritz, and later, Estée Lauder—decorated the faces of women who took their cues from Hollywood stars such as Audrey Hepburn, Grace Kelly, Marilyn Monroe, and Elizabeth Taylor, and from the dictates of American fashion magazines, *Vogue* and *Harper's Bazaar*. The look was one of the prettiest and most sophisticated ever: It was the golden age of the eyebrow, groomed and curved into an amused and worldly "diva arch" that framed the classic doe eye. The fashion magazines adopted the look from the exaggerated eye makeup of the ballet and named it *l'oeil de biche*. The eyes were lined heavily on top with black pencil or liquid liner, which ended in upward wings at the outside corner. Eyelids were decorated with audacious shades of French blue, turquoise, or bottle green, and eyelashes were thickened and lengthened with generous coats of cake mascara. Lips were painted the color of American Beauty roses.

My first memory of paint and powder is of watching my mother apply cosmetics. She said she was "putting on her face," and the transition from "Mama" in her shapeless nightgown to a polished, elegant woman in perfume and high heels was always quite extraordinary.

But my mama would have none of it. Her prohibition against red lipstick was mitigated by substitutes, which in their own way were almost as provocative. I traded in my Tangée Natural for a silvery baby-pink Milkmaid lipstick that smelled of cherry soda and came in a white-enameled, flower-strewn tube. The lipstick was so pale that those of us who wore it resembled snow queens or possibly rosy-cheeked ghosts.

If I became curious about cosmetics watching my mother, my hands-on love affair really started when I was 17. I spent the summer between high school graduation and freshman year of college earning pin money by working as a temporary sales clerk at the large Lazarus department store in my hometown of Columbus, Ohio. Assigned to the cosmetics department, I would rove from counter to counter, selling Elizabeth Arden makeup one day and expensive perfumes the next.

For the magnificent sum of $1.12 an hour, I sold lipstick, mascara, Chanel No. 5, Shalimar, and Arpege. Eventually, I moved to the Revlon counter, where a big day was measured by three or four $25 sales.

To increase traffic at the Revlon counter, Lazarus hired a professional makeup artist whose job was to attract customers by offering free makeovers. The company built a makeup station at the end of the counter with three low stools and installed a very cute guy named Jerry Brandt, who was fresh out of cosmetology school. On slow days, Jerry plopped me down on one of the stools and proceeded to make me up, obliterating my features under a thick layer of pinky-beige foundation. The final touch was always a swipe of Cherries in the Snow, one of Revlon's more vivid and popular shades (Take that, Mama!). In the process, we would draw a crowd that was enthusiastic and curious. Sales were lively.

Charles Revson, a brilliant merchandiser, arrived on the scene at the right time with the right products, although he was often accused by other cosmetics entrepreneurs of stealing formulas and copying trends. Madame Helena Rubinstein called him "that man," and in retaliation, he named his line for men That Man.

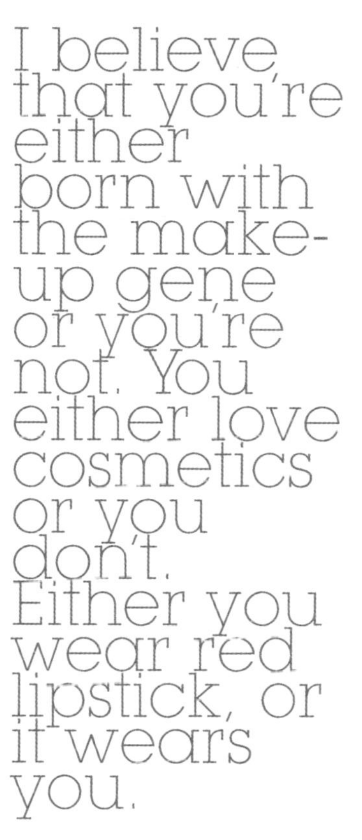
I believe that you're either born with the make-up gene or you're not. You either love cosmetics or you don't. Either you wear red lipstick, or it wears you.

But Charles Revson had killer instincts when it came to merchandising. He perceived that women were ready to paint up and expand their glamour horizons after the deprivations of World War II. With the advent of Technicolor film at the end of the 1930s, makeup became far more natural. Where dark lips had read well in the stylish black-and-white moody film noirs of the late 1930s, a bright, clear red developed for color film that made women look like the "girl next door" became the look prized by American GIs. In the early 1950s Revson intensified the American woman's interest in red lips. The clear red lip color of MGM romantic dramas and musicals became known as MGM Red and was worn by such stars as Marilyn Monroe, Jane Russell, Ann Miller, and Elizbeth Taylor. Such were my icons. And such is the source of my abiding affection for red lipstick.

I believe that you're either born with the makeup gene or you're not. You either love cosmetics or you don't. Either you wear red lipstick, or it wears you. However, there is that safe gray area in between loving makeup and absolutely hating it, where makeup has become a stylistic element essential to the successful career woman or socialite. Many women who would rather spend their days in jeans and sweatshirts with bare, clean faces, sometimes find themselves required to put on a public face while they do business, shop, lunch, or date.

I am not one of those take-it or leave-it females. For me, makeup was and is a joy, not a chore, a fun and fascinating way to recapture my childhood affection for color, play, and "let's pretend."

Even before little girls are old enough to contemplate cosmetics, they fall in love with color. Remember how your heart leapt at the sight of your first box of crayons—pristine cylinders of colored wax, standing like a rainbow of little soldiers, waiting to do your bidding? Remember what it was like to break the crayon in half, peel off the paper, and use it sideways? Remember how your mother taped your crayon masterpieces to the refrigerator? It was a total validation of your imagination and effort.

Mothers through the ages either threw their hands up in disgust, reveled in their daughters' shocking creativity, or didn't care to know about it.

As a child, when you used your crayons, there was no right or wrong. Color was a source of inspiration and fun, a highly disposable expression of personal creativity. It was something that you did every single day in kindergarten. But between kindergarten and first grade, you learned to crayon inside the lines with proper colors. Sky is blue, your teachers said; grass is green. Freedom of expression got educated out of us. Reading, writing, and arithmetic replaced drawing time; art and personal expression were pushed farther into the background. Art class, with its tactile and visual creativity, became an elective instead of an integral part of our studies. Perhaps, in the process, our color muscles atrophied.

The child who loved color became the teenager, subject to peer pressure and parental disapproval. Mom and Dad forbade lipstick, and boyfriends weren't fond of it either. The pack mentality of girlfriends also took over; everyone bought the same color lipstick in an effort to belong. There was comfort in homogeneity; acceptance and security was based on the dictates of our friends.

The process of socialization had one of two effects—it either killed our natural instincts to play with and enjoy color, or it stimulated rebellion. We either conformed to the ideals of our mothers or our peers about what was good and proper makeup, or we continued, psychologically and emotionally, to crayon outside the lines. In the 1950s, girls wore their polite Persian Melon lipstick and very little rouge. In the early 1960s, teenaged girls set their hair around orange-juice cans or ironed it; they blocked out lips with Erase. By the 1980s and 1990s, fashion-curious teens were dying their hair outrageously garish colors, and sneaking off to tattoo wrists, breasts, ankles, or shoulders with butterflies, hearts, soaring birds, or Celtic symbols. Behind their mothers' backs, they pierced bellybuttons and eyebrows, and reveled in colors not found in nature offered by upstart companies like Urban Decay, Rage, or Hard Candy. Their lipstick colors bespoke rebellion: Gas, Flirt, Trailer Trash, Lust, Roach, Asphyxia, Rat, Pleasure/Pain. Mothers through the ages either threw their hands up in disgust, reveled in their daughters' shocking creativity, or didn't care to know about it.

WHY MAKEOVERS USUALLY DON'T WORK

For some of us, cosmetics represent tools of experimentation, personal expression, and pleasure. For others, cosmetics are the requirements of professional life. And for some, they are instruments of intimidation. So how can we explain the overwhelming popularity of the makeover segment of women-hosted afternoon talk shows? Hair, clothing, and makeup professionals select a woman from the audience and change her appearance (not necessarily for the better, by the way). One fashion magazine actually tracks its subjects for a month after their makeovers. It comes as no surprise to me that most of their subjects have gone back to their safe, old styles.

Makeovers can be riveting. We get a vicarious thrill when total strangers transform right before our eyes. At some point, we'll look in the mirror and see the total stranger we've become. Perhaps we'll realize that we are mired in the past, that we're feeling dowdy, that we need a change. When that happens, out of frustration or plain boredom, we'll go to the cosmetics counter and find the young woman painted within an inch of her life and beckoning like Circe: "Would you like to try some of our new colors? Would you like a new look?"

Well, I'm here to tell you that most makeovers do not work. Especially if they're too radical. First of all, the woman behind the counter wants to sell you as much product as possible, particularly if she is working on commission. She wants to give you the latest look according to the corporate makeup artists who have dictated that pink is this season's high-fashion color or that raccoon eyes are cutting-edge fashion. The fact that you look horrendous in pink, that you hate pink, may not even register. In the 15 minutes the department-store makeup artist has you in her chair, is she going to know that you feel more secure with burgundy lipstick and deep, dark eyeliner? Is she going to realize that the sight of red lipstick sends your sweetie into conniptions? Is she going to know that you rub your eyes, and if you wear mascara, you will look like a raccoon by the end of the workday?

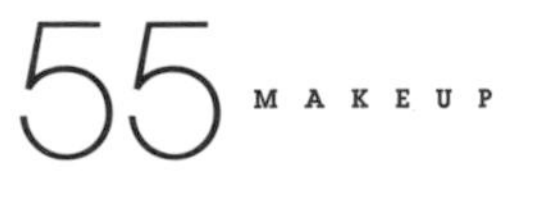

As women, we are continually bombarded with images of perfection against which we are poor contenders.

Probably not. So you could go home with a bag full of makeup that you don't know how to use or that you absolutely hate. Despite all the lessons, the cajoling, and the salesmanship, three months down the road, that bag of makeup will probably sit in a shoe box under your sink—and you'll be back to the look that makes you feel like you.

The word *makeover* implies that there is something wrong with you in the first place; otherwise, why change your look? As women, we are continually bombarded with images of perfection against which we are poor contenders. Slender models, coiffed and painted to perfection by professionals, stare vacantly from magazine covers and advertisements. The obvious message: If you use these products, you too can be slim, gorgeous, loved, adored, adulated, and, yes, envied. I don't think so.

Radical makeovers—where you hair is restyled and colored and your makeup hues are changed—are often difficult and too expensive to maintain. Many times the makeup artist fails to take into consideration that you don't have the time, the budget, or the patience to fuss. But you're contending with a powerfully presented argument: "I am the pro," says the makeup artist. "Trust me. I know how you should look."

Keys to Success

The most successful cosmetic redesigns are the ones that enlist the help of the client in the process. Several times, during promotional appearances in department stores, I've watched makeup artist and cosmetic-company owner Trish McEvoy work with women. She studies the contents of their makeup bags and gains their trust by not telling them that their choices are totally wrong. She asks them several key questions to determine the demands on their time and their attitudes toward cosmetics in general and color in particular. As she goes through the contents of their makeup bags, she keeps what works (and it's more than you'd ever think) and guides them through a reconsideration of other products. She suggests formula and texture updates. She leads the women through a step-by-step makeup lesson; a makeup artist does half the client's face, then the client takes over the brushes and colors

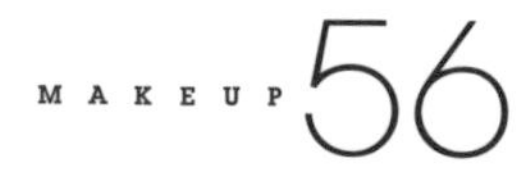

and finishes the look under the careful eye of the makeup artist. This results in a communicative partnership between makeup artist and client.

Purchasing Makeup

The process of purchasing makeup can be intimidating. I don't know how many women have sighed in exasperation and said, "I hate to shop." Liberally translated, that phrase becomes fraught with meaning: "I hate having people look at me critically while I'm buying a lipstick." "I feel less than acceptable because I don't look like the pictures of the glamorous young models at the counter." "I'm afraid I'll buy the wrong thing."

Remember, there is only one hard and fast rule: *You do not have to buy a single thing*. For your first foray, go to the counter with no money or credit cards in your pocket so that when you say, "I'm just looking," you mean it.

Regardless of why you go to the cosmetic counter, control your own experience. Be willing to experiment; be open to what the counter person has to say to you, but communicate with her. Talk about your likes and dislikes, the demands on your time, and your budget. Remember, you do not have to buy anything, but if you have your makeup done, you've taken up the time of a professional, so it's only polite to spend some money in exchange for her time and expertise. But don't be forced by a misplaced sense of obligation to buy *everything*. A lipstick or a mascara will do.

Take advantage of a company's liberal sampling program of skincare products, packets of foundation, or teensy mascaras. Ask for moisturizers and eye creams to try at home, and once you've found one you can live with, go back and invest in it. Chances are, if you buy products that you use, you'll be back. And that's what the cosmetic companies really want: repeat business.

Developing Your Own Signature Look

We all have our favorite colors that resonate emotionally—hues that make us feel good, that define who we are. Regardless of how uncomplimentary they are to our skin tone or how dated they look, we are reluctant to give them up. At some point, certain aspects of makeup can become signatures, or even life rafts—like Elizabeth Taylor's heavy mascara and violet eyeshadow

Regardless of why you go to the cosmetic counter, control your own experience. Be willing to experiment.

Maybe it's time to measure your attitude and preconceptions about cosmetics.

or Cindy Crawford's mole, which she does not hide under concealer. Or Tammy Faye Bakker's spidery fake eyelashes. To ask her to remove them would be like asking her to amputate an arm. Those eyelashes *are* Tammy Faye.

In the early 1990s, when Tammy Faye and her then-under-indictment husband, Jim, were in San Francisco conferring with their lawyer, Melvin Belli, someone had the great idea of taking Tammy Faye to a prominent local salon to have her makeup redone. It was an attempt to give her a quieter style, so she would be taken seriously by the court and by her critics, who focused on her makeup mistakes: heavy, pearlized eye shadow, overdrawn mouth, and eyebrows redrawn over her natural ones. And, oh yes, those lashes.

Coreen Cordova, the makeup artist assigned to work on Tammy Faye, asked her why she had made her cosmetic choices. Tammy Faye said, "Because I want to look as cute and cuddly as a Kewpie doll." Coreen replied, "How could I argue with that?"

WHAT KIND OF MAKEUP PERSON ARE YOU?

Before you even set foot inside a department store and attempt to fathom the hundreds of products calling out to you to buy them, you'll have to ask yourself: *How do I feel about makeup? Do I like the way it smells and feels? Do I know how to use it? Do I feel foolish wearing it?* Maybe it's time to measure your attitude and preconceptions about cosmetics.

Let's play a little game. Answer the questions in the following lists to see if you are makeup phobic, moderately curious, a makeup casualty, a makeup addict, or a makeup diva. If you answer yes to a majority of the questions in any of these very arbitrary categories, then the shoe fits, but you don't necessarily have to wear it forever. Your answers will give you an indication of how you feel about wearing makeup and why you've made the choices you have. From there, it's easy to modify your behavior.

Are You Makeup Phobic?

- **Are you an adult who has never owned mascara?**
- **Are you unsure how to use blush or where to put it?**
- **Have you always thought that women who wear makeup are vain and shallow?**
- **Do makeup counters scare you?**
- **Do you think lipstick makes you look cheap?**
- **Are you unsure how to buy foundation?**
- **Do you avoid using moisturizer?**
- **Are you stymied by the terms *AHA* and *BHA*?**

Interpretation.

If you've answered yes to at least three of these questions, there is a good chance that for some reason, makeup has no part in your life. But you find yourself faced with a problem: You're getting older and your skin is starting to show it. Perhaps you've been out in the sun with inadequate protection; maybe you're of Scotch-English extraction and your already delicate skin is getting dry and thin. Maybe you are a reentry woman, back in the job market after raising a family. For whatever reason, your life is requiring that you put your best face forward and you don't know how.

Are You a Diva In Training?

- **Do you read fashion magazines and look at the ads?**
- **Have you ever wanted to have a makeover or a makeup lesson?**
- **Have you ever made a totally out-of-character impulse purchase of a red lipstick or glitter nail polish?**
- **Do you admire women whose makeup is always perfect?**
- **Did you ever spend a half hour in a drugstore playing with makeup testers?**
- **Do you wander through cosmetic departments, window shopping and trying perfume?**
- **Have you ever shut the door to your bathroom, made up your face, and then washed it off immediately?**
- **Have you ever looked at yourself in the mirror, acknowledged that you needed a change, but then shrugged your shoulders and forgotten about it?**

Interpretation.

How does this sample scenario fit? Perhaps you've spent most of your adult years taking care of a home and children; maybe you've been in graduate school or you haven't had the cash to spend on a total look. You've had hardly any privacy or time for yourself, so some things have slid—like putting on lipstick, mascara, and blusher. Any attempts you've made at staking out your own time and space have been interrupted by insistent clients wanting something sent out immediately, or by a teenager who stays in the bathroom for hours primping, or by young children who haven't quite learned the intricacies of privacy (nothing like luxuriating in your bath, only to have your two-year-old stumble in with a full diaper).

But say you've always wanted to look better, to present an image to the world that says you're in control and that you care about yourself. You've just not had the time or energy to do it. All of which means, you're probably a good candidate for some creative changes and maybe even a makeup lesson. You're willing to take the time, now that you have it, to learn how to put your best face forward.

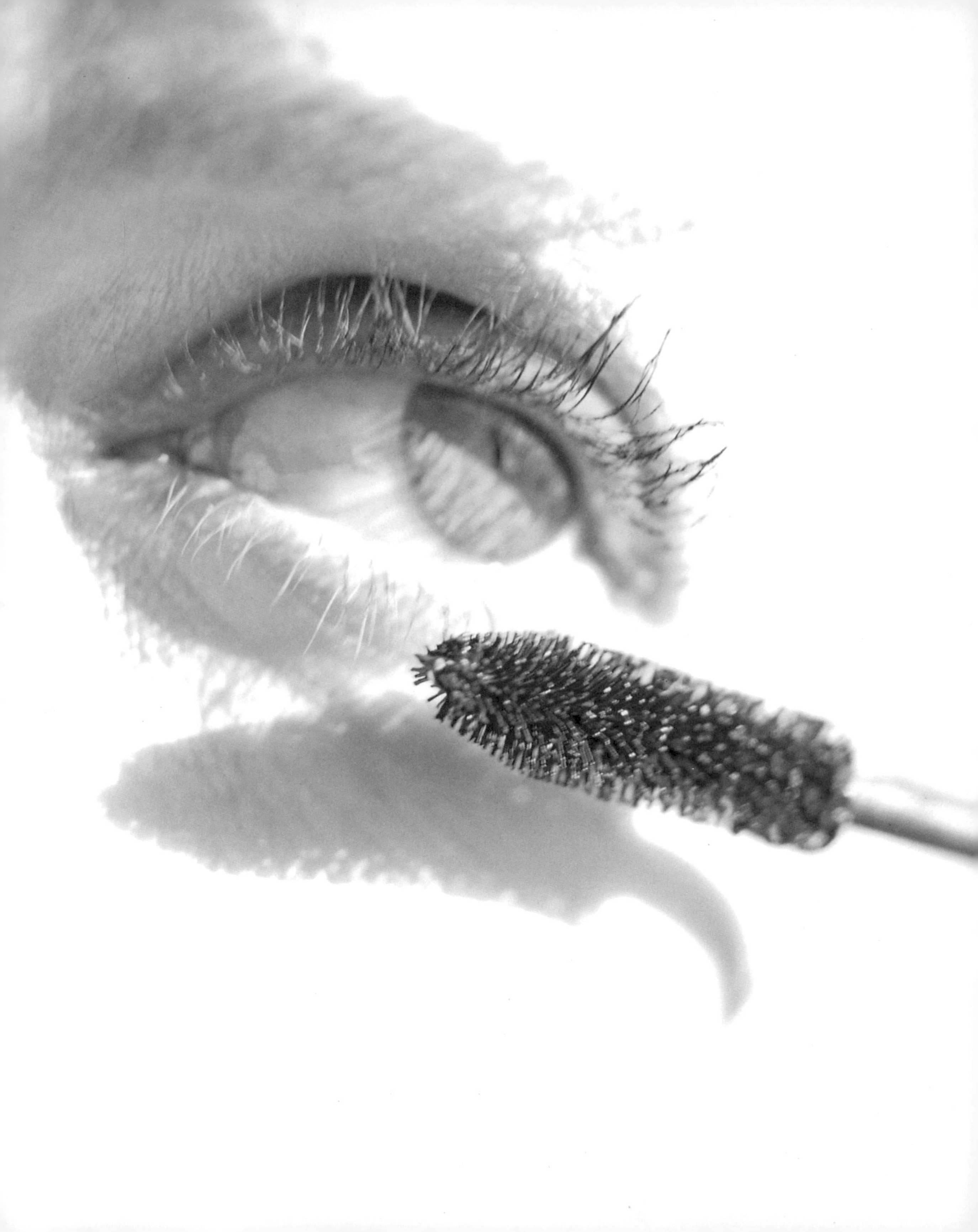

Are You Trapped in a Cosmetic Time Warp?

- *Have you worn the same lipstick since graduating from high school or college?*
- *Do you have a signature scent from which you never vary?*
- *Are you wearing your hair the same way you did five years ago?*
- *Are you trying to duplicate the look you had when you thought you looked your best and felt the most confident?*
- *Are you devastated and stymied when you learn that your favorite makeup colors have been discontinued?*
- *Do you cling to certain cosmetics like a lifeline despite the fact that eye shadows have changed radically and that liver-colored matte lips date you?*
- *When your friends give you something new to try, do you toss it in the back of your makeup drawer and forget about it?*

Interpretation.

If these questions resonate with you and you've answered most of them with a yes, you do not like change; it makes you uncomfortable. Ask yourself this: *Am I too scared to try something new because I already know how to do what I'm doing? Am I afraid of making a mistake and looking stupid? Or am I just lazy?* Maybe you aren't aware that the makeup you're using is dated. Maybe your significant other likes you the way you are, and you don't want to rock the boat. Maybe there is so much stuff out there that making a choice is daunting. You have an inkling that you need a change, but you've really stopped looking at yourself in the mirror. Putting on the same old stuff day after day has become rote. It's a routine you know, but you're afraid of what you don't know. You are ripe for an update.

Are You a Makeup Addict?

- Do you know the names of more than one superstar makeup artist? Do the names Kevin Aucoin, Mary Greenwell, François Nars, Vincent Longo, Jeanine Lobell, Bobbi Brown, Carol Shaw, or Laura Mercier ring a bell?
- Are you always changing your look to coincide with current fashion trends?
- Do you subscribe to *W, Vogue, Harper's Bazaar, Elle,* and/ or *Allure*?
- Do you have unopened boxes and bottles of cosmetics stored in your linen closet?
- Do you own more than 10 lipsticks?
- Do you have mascara in more than two colors?
- Do you rush out and buy the new colors from more than one cosmetic line each season?
- Do you ever go to cosmetic counters for a makeover and end up buying everything in the line?
- Are you uncomfortable leaving your house with anything less than full makeup?
- Are you uncomfortable letting anyone (including the UPS delivery person) see you without makeup?

Interpretation.

Your deep and abiding affection for make-up has much to do with whether you were encouraged to use it when you were young or forbidden to do so by a strict parent. You could be a total fool for color—your heart races (a classic addictive symptom, psychologists will tell you) when you walk into a cosmetic department and are facing myriad choices for purchase. You could be an outgoing, exhibitionistic person who will be noticed, who will not be ignored. Or you can be putting on a public face and being more out there than you'd be without makeup. In any event, less is not more for you.

There is probably no cure for your cosmetic addiction or your hunger for newness and change. What you need is a steady, guiding influence to teach you how to limit the products you put on your face to the ones that will show off your natural assets to best advantage. Ask yourself this: *Can I throw out the contents of my makeup drawer, buy only what I need to enhance my face, and forget about the rest?* If the answer is yes, then do it. Otherwise, enjoy playing. When it comes to makeup, regardless of what other people think or what your conformist instincts tell you, *there is no right or wrong, if it makes you feel good.* But . . . a little editing couldn't harm you.

Are you uncomfortable letting anyone (including the UPS delivery person) see you without makeup?

Are You a Makeup Diva?

- Do you own more than three lipsticks but fewer than six?
- Do you update your look with a new color or texture every season?
- Are you comfortable trying something new at the suggestion of a friend or because you read about it in a magazine?
- Do you regularly have your makeup done for special occasions?
- Do you feel undressed or unfinished without lipstick and mascara?
- Can you do your makeup in under 15 minutes and walk out the door feeling secure?

Interpretation.

Chances are you love color and aren't afraid to use it. You could be in a high-profile job where you travel and meet people constantly, and the underlying message from your company is to look more than just presentable—to be confident and even glamorous. You could be married to a man whose business demands that the two of you be very social. Your mother may have taken you in hand and shared her beauty secrets. You may have received positive reinforcement from the men and boys in your life when you wore a pretty dress or blusher, polished your nails, or put on lipstick.

If you're a makeup diva, you're not afraid of what cosmetics can do with and for you. You'll probably never overdo it because cosmetics have taken their natural place in your life—as enhancement not crutch. You can control them, and you love playing with them.

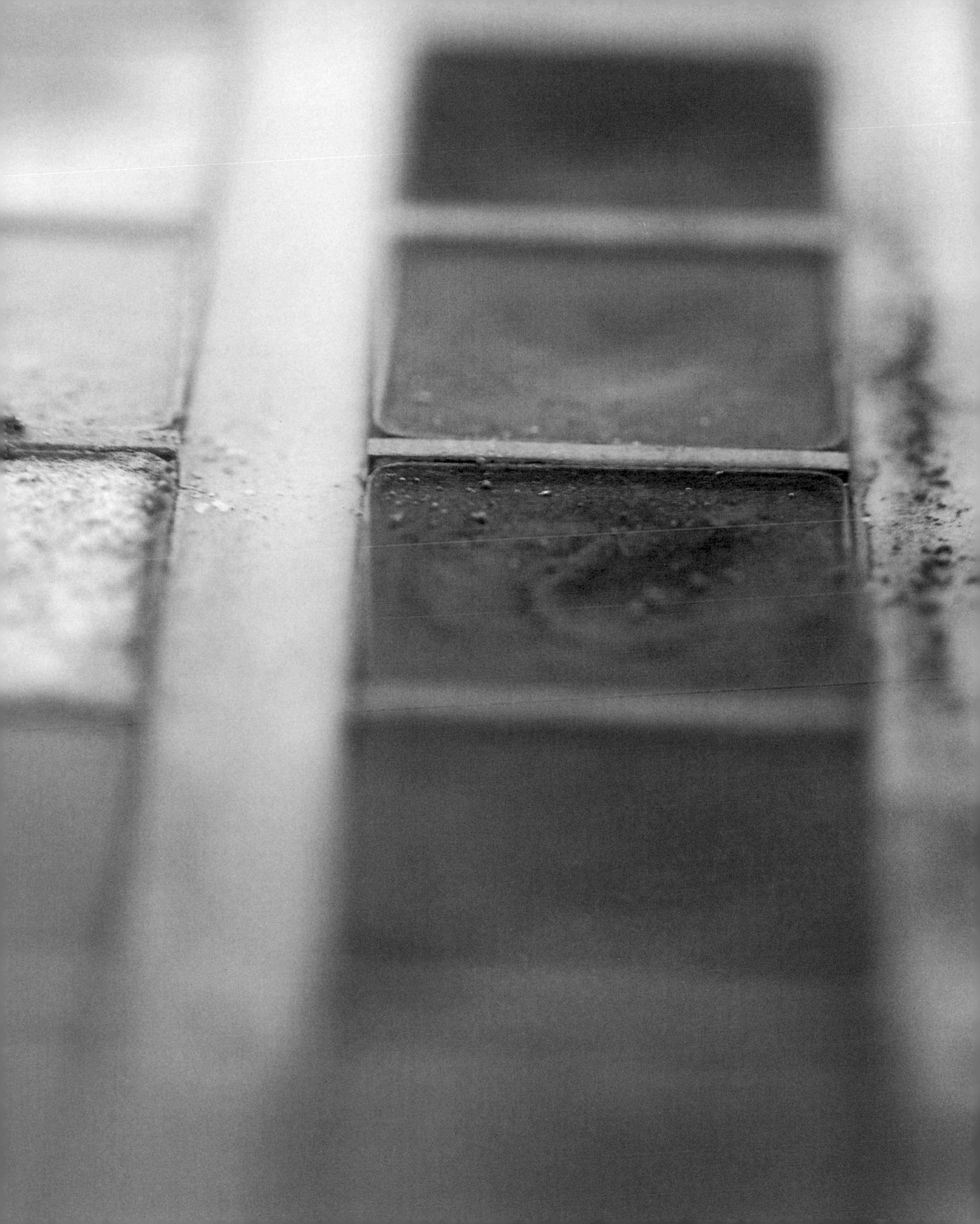

Personal Best

My goal for you is to help you develop your inner comfort level about cosmetics. As smart makeup artists who have you in their chair will do, you've got to ask yourself the right questions to find out how far you can go. What do you want from makeup? A finished, well-groomed look that exudes self-confidence? An ego-boosting experience? An escape—the ability to become someone else entirely? Whatever your motives, the bottom line is: *Makeup is fun.*

Starting Fresh with Your Inner Makeup Diva

1. Take an inventory of your current supply of makeup. Decide what you can live without, and throw out what you can.
2. Have a cosmetic consultation, but do it with a makeup artist who will give you a lesson as he or she works on your face.
3. Buy a lipstick or an eye shadow whose color attracts you, one that you have not bought before. Take it home and wear it around the house to get comfortable with it before taking it to the street.
4. Practice, practice, practice in front of your mirror. Remember, there is no right or wrong way to do things, just the way that works for you.
5. Makeup is not a permanent commitment. You can wash off your mistakes.
6. Have fun.

GETTING TO KNOW YOUR OWN FACE.

Women are creatures of habit. We stare into the mirror first thing in the morning and what does our eye immediately focus on? Not a voluptuous lip but the cold sore in the corner of it. Not a noble nose but a zit developing on the tip. Not clear, lucid blue eyes with golden haloes, but the dark circles and new pouches beneath. And those teensy lines around our eyes that seem to have come out of nowhere.

In other words, we look at ourselves and see the worst. No wonder when it comes to putting on makeup, we do it wrong. Instead of focusing on, enhancing, and highlighting our best features, we try to hide, obscure, negate, obliterate, mask, and cover what we perceive as our facial faults.

I'd like you to play a couple of games that can alter your perception of how you look.

Stranger-in-the-Mirror Game

① Stand before your bathroom mirror and close your eyes before you have a chance to look at yourself. Take a deep breath.

② Open your eyes quickly and pretend the face looking back at you belongs to a total stranger, someone you are meeting for the first time.

③ Give your image a compliment. (Haven't our mothers always told us to find something nice to say about somebody when we meet them?)

④ Be quick and instinctual about it. Don't look at that image and go to the same old, tired territory of self-criticism. Be nice. Just like your mama told you.

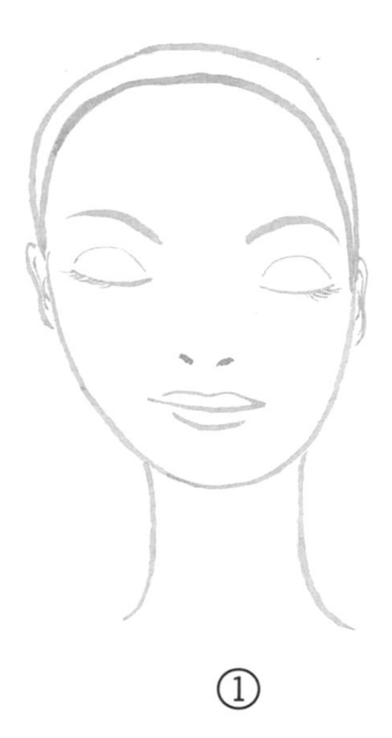

①

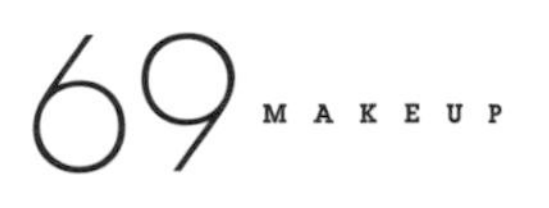

Interpretation.

Be prepared for a couple of things to happen here. First of all, you'll be amazed at what comes out of your mouth if you've been spontaneous. You will start to notice the positive aspects of your face—the color of your eyes, the curve of your eyebrows, the prominence of your cheekbones. These are the building blocks of your face, the features that deserve enhancement.

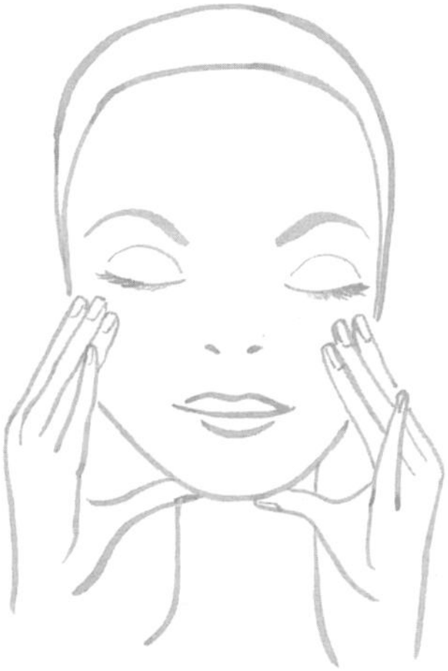

Face Game

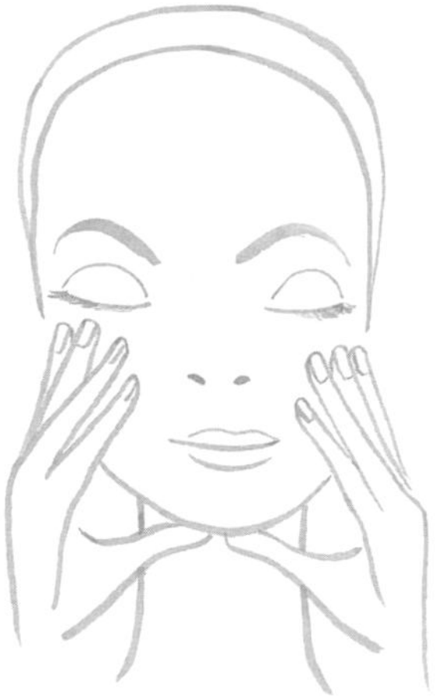

① Pick a time when you know you will not be disturbed and lock yourself in the bathroom.

② Pin your hair away from your face.

③ Wash your hands carefully and turn out the light (or simply close your eyes). No cheating here. You're going to do this game with your fingers, not your eyes.

④ With your thumbs hooked solidly under your chin, allow your fingers to uncurl naturally over your cheeks. What do you feel? Your cheekbones, right?

⑤ Walk your fingers gently back along each cheekbone from its point closest to your nose to its apex, where it curves down toward your ear.

⑥ Turn on the light and look into the mirror. Place your hands back on your face in the same manner (thumbs hooked under chin, fingers curled naturally and resting on your cheekbones). Trace the apex of your cheekbone and smile. Is the fullest part of your cheek when you're smiling at the apex of your cheekbone? That's called the apple of your cheek, and it is the best place to put blusher.

⑦ Turn off the light again and proceed to your mouth. With the fourth finger of your hand, the ring finger, gently trace the outline of your lips. Are your lips bigger than you thought they were? Can you feel a ridge at the outside edge? That ridge is going to be the border for lip liner and lip color. By coloring inside the ridge, you can reduce the size of larger lips; by lining directly on or slightly outside the ridge, you can make your lips appear bigger.

⑧ Now it's time to examine your eyes. Close them gently. Do not squint. With your index finger or your ring finger, feel the area on the upper lid, from the lash line to right under the occipital bone, or eye socket. In the simplest, most neutral makeups, this is where you will brush on eyeshadow.

⑨ Tilt your head down and allow your chin to rest gently on your chest. Now, arch your eyebrows with great exaggeration and trace the brow on its upward curve. Place your finger at the highest point and let your brows relax. This is your eyebrow arch. The area right under it is where highlighter eye shadow goes.

⑩ Now place your hand in a vertical position, running alongside your nose to your eyebrow. If you can feel any eyebrow hairs on the side of that finger nearest the nose, they probably need to be tweezed away.

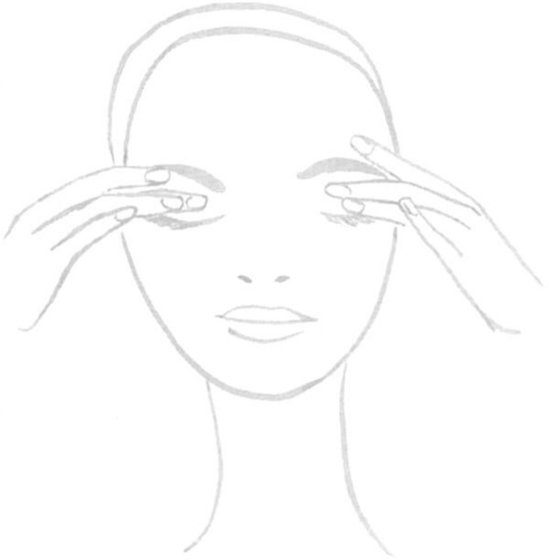

⑧

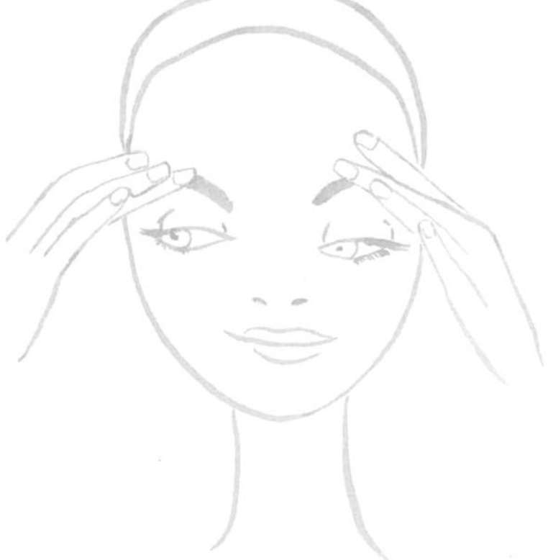

⑨

Repeat all of the above exercises in the light, noting where the landmarks of your face are and the areas I have suggested for makeup. You do not need to determine the shape of your face—whether it is triangular, heart-shaped, oval, square, or round—to apply makeup. By locating the monuments of your own facial topography, you'll have a map for simple, flattering makeup.

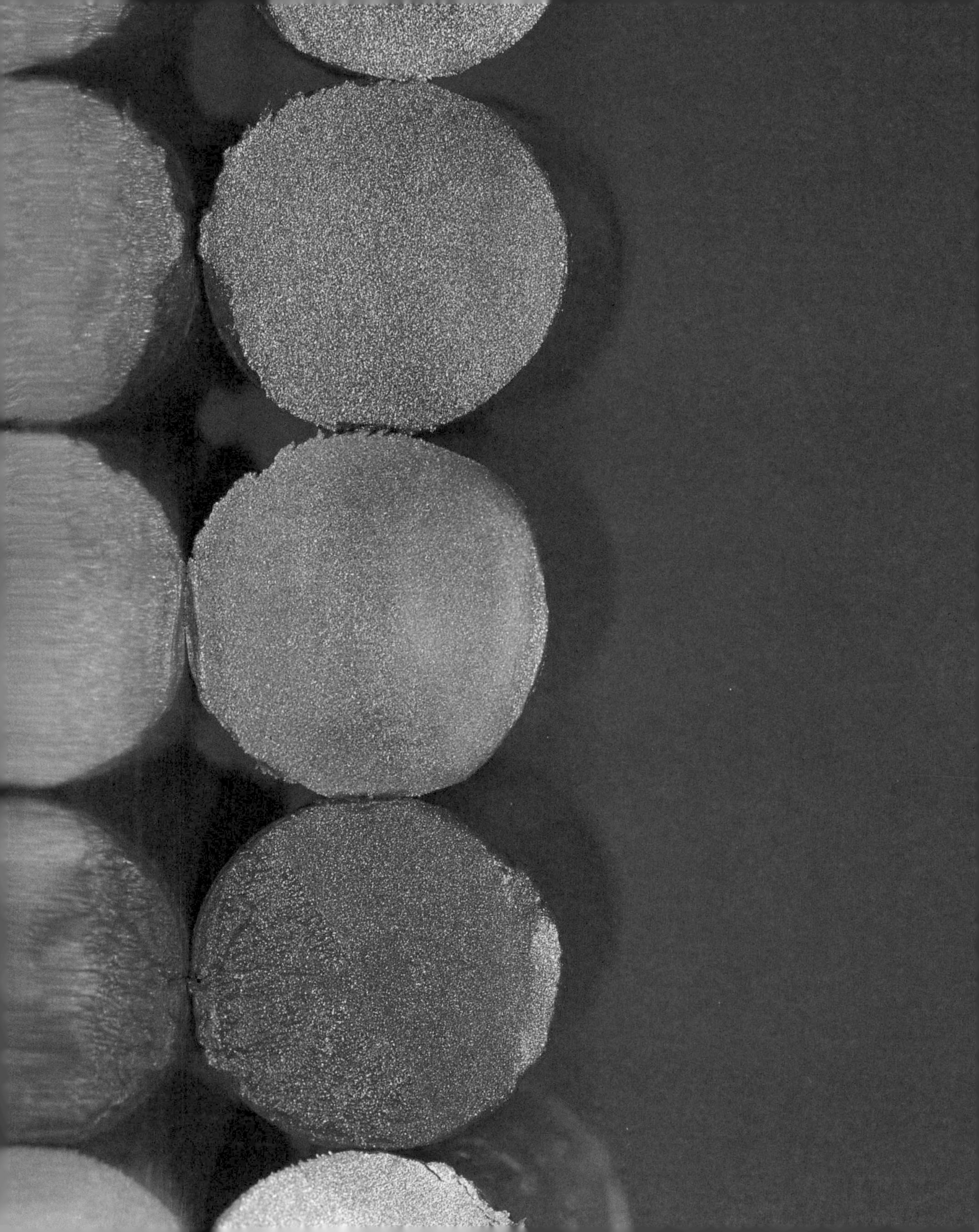

Solving the Mystery of Color Choice

There are no hard-and-fast rules about what colors you should use. It's not very complicated: If you like it, wear it. And if you don't like it, don't wear it. There is one proviso, however: If a makeup artist or clothing consultant has suggested that you wear a color that has never been in your makeup kit or wardrobe before, don't just dismiss it. Maybe that color is most complimentary to your own coloring. Maybe it accents your eyes or makes your skin glow. Perhaps it turns up the volume on your personal charisma. Do not automatically reject that color. First, consider these questions: *Why don't I like this color? What does it remind me of? What is the root of my fear and prejudice?*

As adults, the colors we prefer are the ones that have been reinforced by early conditioning, either by positive or negative comments. Because my own mother hated bright colors, I wear them today—vivid shades like red, orange, and kelly green. My mother was a very quiet, shy woman who was concerned about propriety, and in the 1950s she was a proper housewife and mother. She dressed very conservatively in navy blue, beige, and celadon green. I don't think she ever owned a pink blouse or a purple sweater in her life. She attempted to form me in her image, but I hated beige and navy, and wear very little, if any, of those colors as an adult. When I was old enough to buy my own clothes and cosmetics, I rebelled. My closet is filled with black, white, and red clothes, none of which my mother would have worn herself.

You might want to ask yourself: *Am I wearing a color I've worn since childhood? Or am I dressed in something my mother would have hated?* Chances are, if you were praised as a child when you had on a frilly pink dress, black Mary Janes, and socks with blue flowers, these are the colors that you cherish today.

Leatrice Eiseman, a color psychologist and author of *Colors for Your Every Mood*, says that how we feel about color is embedded in our unconscious "until or unless we let other people disapprove or lend their own opinions based on their own color prejudices." If you allow yourself to listen to the opinions of too many people, you could, she says, "dilute your own intrinsic and inherent feelings about color."

Color is, first and foremost, an emotional issue. Colors that we love and would never abandon remind us of things that once happened in our lives.

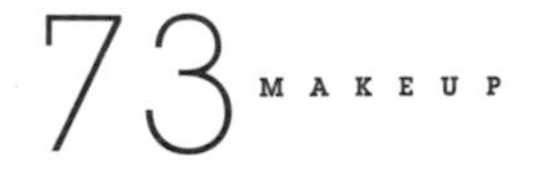

Color is, first and foremost, an emotional issue. Colors that we love and would never abandon remind us of things that once happened in our lives. Maybe a favorite pink or peach was the color of a prom dress or the ribbon on our confirmation gown. By wearing it, we will always be in touch, in some tactile, real-world way, with the emotions the color recalls.

Color as a tool for rebellion starts when children need to distinguish themselves from their parents' generation. For this reason alone, it's easy to understand why a bank president's daughter will dye her hair bright green or paint her nails black. Our color choices also come from wanting to please the people we love and respect. Sometimes we give away too much of our ability to choose for ourselves. Because we are aware of the preferences of our loved ones, we put them before our own choices if we are insecure or don't want an argument.

There are ways of reaching compromises with the loved ones in your life. If red lips are definitely out or green eyeshadow is a no-no regardless of how emerald it makes your eyes look, then bring home three other colors you love, model them, and choose the compromise colors together.

Color-Q Test

As socialized grown-ups, we should ask ourselves whether our ingrained attitudes about color have changed over the years or whether they are candidates for change now. What if, for instance, your best friend who thinks you'd look smashing in peach gave you a peach blouse—but you've never even thought of wearing that color? Can you put it on and see yourself through her eyes? Do you feel buoyant, attractive, pretty, comfortable?

What if you needed to refresh your lipstick and you forgot to put one in your bag before you left home? Your friend offers to lend you hers but it's a color—let's say a strong brown/red—that you would never choose for yourself. Do you say, "No thank you, I won't wear any," or will you try it? You may be surprised by what other people have to say about it, but it's your opinion that should take precedence. Look in the mirror. How does the new color make you feel? Does it brighten up your face? Make your lips seem fuller? Does it make your eye color pop? Maybe by using your friend's lipstick, you'll discover something different about yourself: that the lipstick gives you confidence and that you actually like it.

In the next few pages, you are going to learn about your color likes and dislikes when it comes to traditional makeup shades. Look at the color chart on the following page. The lipstick colors are popular shades ranging from neutrals and polite pinks and mauves to hot corals, reds, and vampy burgundies. The eyeshadows are fairly standard colors that you can find in just about every cosmetic line. Chart your reaction to each color: Do you love it? Do you like it? Do you dislike it? Do you positively hate it? Write your reaction beside the color.

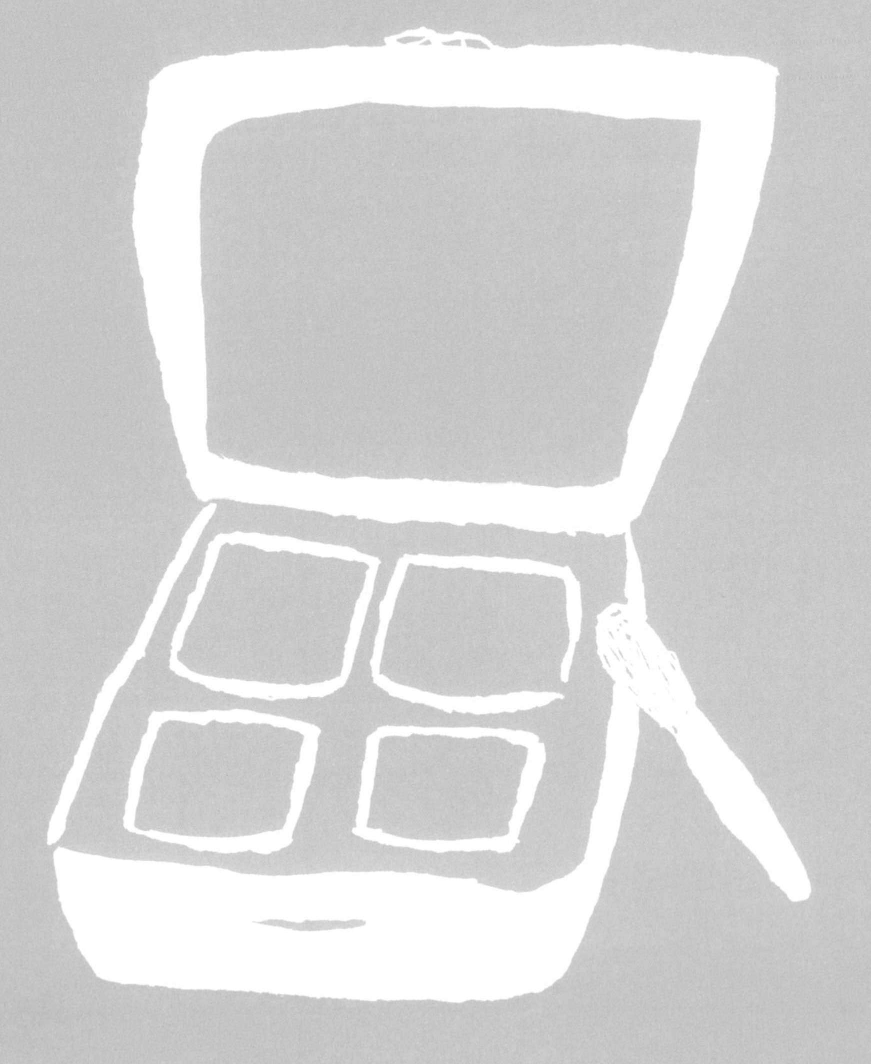

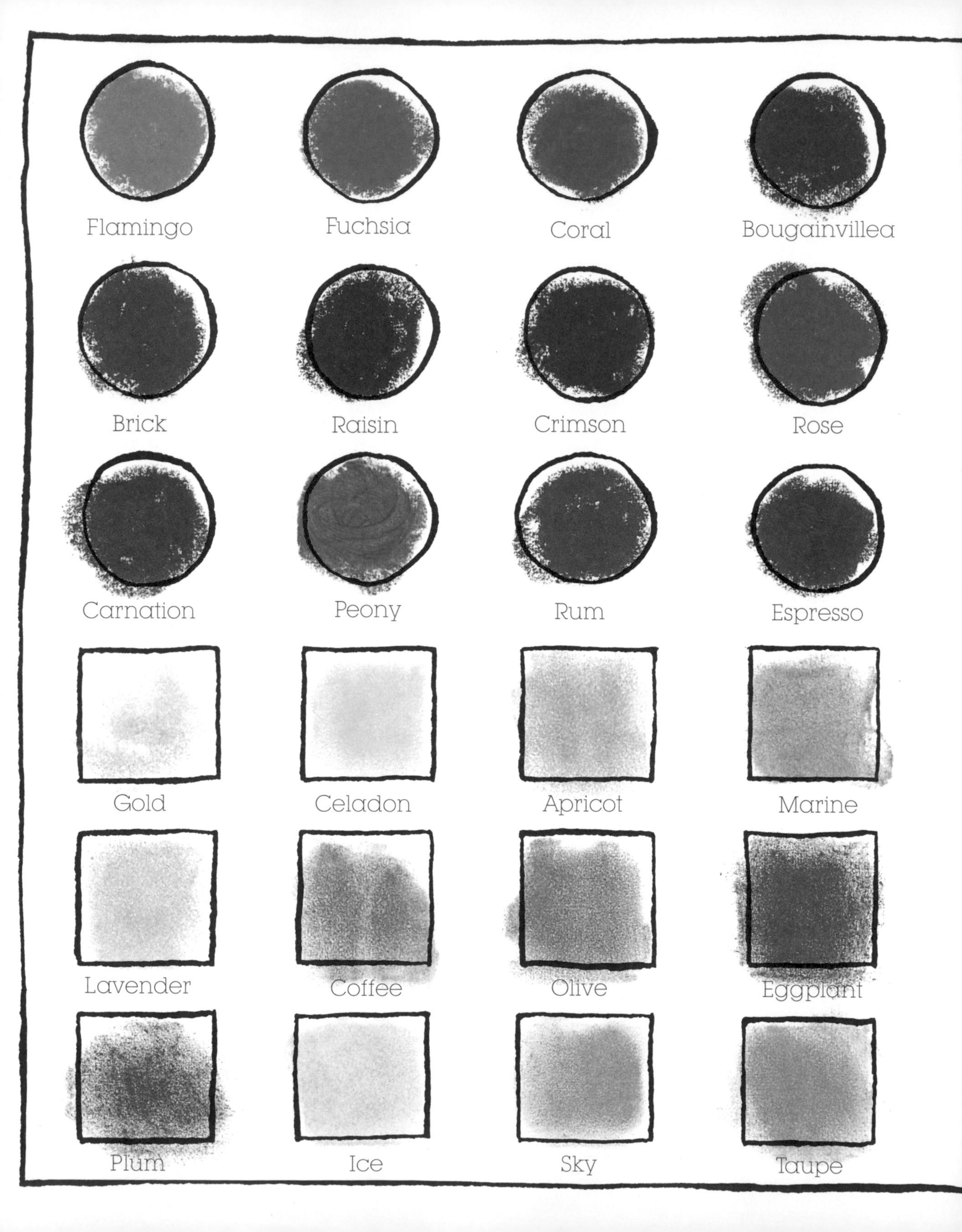
Flamingo
Fuchsia
Coral
Bougainvillea
Brick
Raisin
Crimson
Rose
Carnation
Peony
Rum
Espresso
Gold
Celadon
Apricot
Marine
Lavender
Coffee
Olive
Eggplant
Plum
Ice
Sky
Taupe

My Color Attitude

Now look at each color a second time and find words to describe your feelings about it:

① **I like this color because it is:**
- Inviting • Nurturing • Friendly • Stimulating • Traditional • Classy
- Sensual • Approachable • Dynamic • Neutral • Tasteful • Pretty

② **I do not like this color because it is:**
- Disturbing • Disgusting • Insipid • Tough • Ugly
- Nauseating • Blah • Glaring • Insipid • Weak • Sterile
- Harsh • Dull • Noisy • Artificial • Tasteless

③ **This color makes me feel:**
- Hot • Cool • Sterile • Cold • Uncomfortable • Relaxed • Flirty
- Sophisticated • Sad • Weak • Traditional • Neutral • Beautiful

④ **This color reminds me of something:**
- Masculine • Feminine • Powerful • Cheap • Spiritual
- Serious • Mysterious • Garish

⑤ **If I wore this color I would feel:**
- Powerful • Tasteful • Sexy • Romantic • Approachable
- Artificial • Unfriendly • Bland • Sad • Ugly • Peaceful
- Beautiful • Strong • Passionate • Elegant • Dirty
- Obvious • Rich

⑥ **This color may be good for me because it is:**
- Warm • Cool • Neutral • Striking • Sunny • Inviting
- Earthy • Subtle

⑦ **I am attracted to this color for its:**
- Passion • Directness • Stimulation • Tranquility • Sweetness
- Mystery • Fun

This exercise, developed by Leatrice Eiseman, will help you define why some colors please you and others turn you off. A willingness to experiment may open your mind and broaden your personal color spectrum. For instance, if the coral lipstick made you giggle and your reaction was, "Love it but would not wear it," maybe you should reconsider and try it. Buy a coral lipstick. Try it on in the privacy of your bathroom. Wear it around the house when no one is there or when you are home in your sweats on a Saturday or Sunday. See how you feel in it. Then wear it out and see how other people react to you in it. You may have discovered that you're not a mocha/neutral kind of gal, after all, and that the coral lipstick gives you confidence, brightens your face, and injects some harmless fun into your life.

Best Face Forward: Makeup and How to Use It

Many women ask, "Why wear makeup?" And to them, I say, "Why not?" Cosmetics are tools, used to help you put your best face forward, whether you simply slick on a lip gloss, brush your eyebrows, and walk out the door or put on full "war paint." The goal is to enhance your public face.

What does a finished face say about you? That you've taken some time. That you care about yourself. That you have self-confidence. That you're not ashamed of looking pretty or glamorous or fresh or even adorable. I use the word *finished* a lot in this book. To me, it means that you've polished off the rough edges to present a complete portrait. *Finished*, however, does not mean *done*, as in: She spent hours on her makeup and it looks like it. Makeup, if applied with a light, sure hand, compliments. A good makeup is one in which you, and not your makeup, are noticed.

I've always said that if you have to spend more than 10 minutes in front of your mirror with your makeup, don't bother. You're probably using too much. If you look like you've worked too hard on your face, it sends messages that you probably don't want anyone to receive: that you're insecure, too concerned with your appearance, want to be noticed, and are allowing your makeup to speak for you. Whatever the reason, too much makeup is probably worse than none at all–people will see your makeup, not you.

So what is the purpose of cosmetics? What are the messages you want to impart? That you are self-caring, not conceited. That you are conscientious, not obsessed. That you are finished, not done.

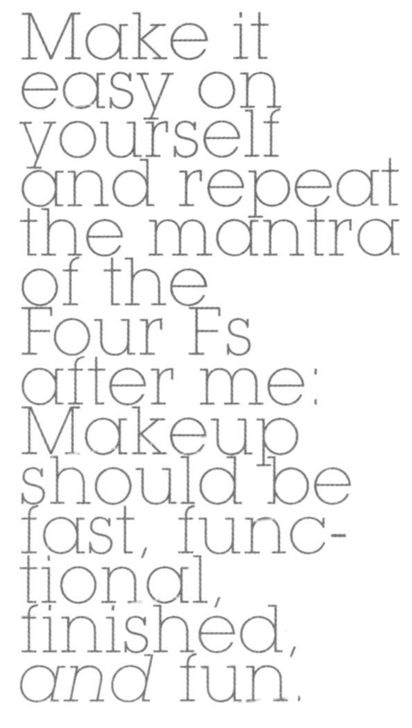
Make it easy on yourself and repeat the mantra of the Four Fs after me: Makeup should be fast, functional, finished, *and* fun.

There are few rules when it comes to wearing makeup. Mostly, though, makeup should be about easy technique and personal taste.

- Once you know the topography of your face, you'll know where to apply makeup.
- Once you've become adept at putting on cosmetics (practice, practice, practice), you should be able to do it in less than 10 minutes.
- Once you know what you're doing, you can start having fun.

MAKEUP TRENDS

Sometimes it's easier to get professional help when you're just beginning to wear cosmetics or when you want to change your look. Make sure that when you sit down at a cosmetic counter for a redo, you tell the makeup artist *exactly* what your goals are, whether you'd just like a new foundation or you want a totally fresh look. A good makeup artist will work with you, not against you.

You can also go and have your makeup done just to see if the season's latest colors will work on you. (You can always wash them off when you get home.) Trendy colors, however, are usually designed for single-season wear. They are chosen each season when makeup artists ask designers what colors they want to use on the runway. In the case of designers such as Karl Lagerfeld of Chanel and Yves Saint Laurent, the seasonal makeup *colorways*, as they are called, derive directly from that season's haute couture collection.

Sometimes trendy runway colors are downright silly (like Betsey Johnson's poison green eye shadow one season). Karl Lagerfeld's pronouncement that he wanted his models to have smeared eye makeup, as if "they'd been up all night," is an example of a runway look that will rarely translate into the language of commercial beauty products.

The Infamous Vamp

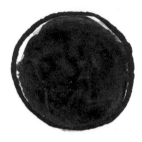

Once in a while, a color meant solely for the runway will become a runaway favorite. Such was Chanel's radical black-burgundy nail polish (and later a lipstick) called Vamp. It was the color of dried blood and wasn't intended as anything more than a runway accent color for the Chanel's Spring 1994 couture collection. But after the fashion press got a look at it, it became a phenomenon that eventually revived Chanel's flagging nail polish business. When style-conscious women who buy couture and those who closely follow press reports out of Paris heard about this unusual new shade, they had to have it. Chanel's marketing team swung into action and rushed the color into production. By the time it was on the cosmetic counter in June 1994, it was already a cultural phenomenon. A color superstar.

Chanel designer Karl Lagerfeld had originally intended to paint his model's nails black for a photo shoot, but then got the idea that a blood-red-black polish would look chic with his pastel spring collection. The original black nails were created from water-soluble black paint. After many tries in the lab at combining black and red, brown and burgundy, rose and black, Vamp was developed.

All the trendy women wanted to be the first on their block to have nails the color of Dracula's favorite beverage. Stories came out of Beverly Hills and New York that counter clerks at Bloomingdale's and Barney's were offered as much as $100 to hand over their tester bottles. Actress Faye Dunaway sent her limousine driver into a Rodeo Drive boutique to borrow the Vamp tester to take to her manicurist. Her driver returned the bottle when Dunaway's fingernails were properly painted.

So what was the big deal? Black-hued nail polishes had been popular, albeit with punk girls and rock stars, for years. Iggy Pop wore black nails. So did Joan Jett. But Vamp obviously struck a chord, and it crossed all age and class boundaries. High school girls adored it and were willing to pay nearly $15 for the real deal. Wealthy society women flocked to it in droves. Vamp was a way for them to rock out without seeming too impolite. If they were wearing Chanel and Karl Lagerfeld had designed it, what could be so improper about Vamp?

From that single nail color, Chanel created a fashion that women were reluctant to give up until nearly six years later, when nails and lips returned to a traditional bright red. But Vamp spawned a franchise: Vamp mascara, lipstick, and polish. Obviously, women embraced Vamp wholeheartedly, making it an instant classic. That phenomenon is rare. Most of the time, fashion colors are as ephemeral as snow in Atlanta. They are designed to disappear almost as quickly as they arrive.

TOOLS OF THE TRADE

Let us suppose, then, that you have been to the store and you have a new bag of makeup that you can't wait to try. How are you going to use it?

First of all you need the proper implements—brushes, sponges, velour puffs, cotton swabs, pencil sharpeners, and eyelash curlers—that will transfer what is in the pot, tube, compact, and bottle to your face with the correct consistency and vibrancy. Then you will need to know what you've got, how to use it, and where to put it.

The best tools in your arsenal are you fingers. You've already used them to discover the landmarks on your face. With them, you will be able to accomplish a natural-looking makeup—that is, if you use them lightly and delicately. And of course, cleanly. If you plan to put your fingers into pots of foundation or cream blusher, make sure your hands are clean, because you can transfer bacteria to these instant, culture mediums. There, microscopic nasties can grow and prosper and come back to haunt you with irritations, clogged pores, and breakouts. You can also apply makeup with an assortment of common implements found in drugstores.

Sponge. Foundations applied with a sponge look soft and sheer; sponges blend better than fingers do. Sponges should be thrown away after one or two uses.

Velour Powder Puff. A washable tool for blending the edges of your foundation and blusher, a velour puff gives your foundation a very soft, sheer appearance.

Beauty Tip 01: Old, soft toothbrushes make great eyebrow brushes.

Cotton Swab. Keep two-ended swabs handy for applying small amounts of moisturizer and foundation or for neatening up mascara, eyeliner, and lipstick.

Pencil Sharpener. To keep your eyebrow, eyeliner, and lip-liner pencils sharpened, you'll need two or three sizes of sharpeners to match your arsenal of pencils.

Eyelash Curler. Use one to curl your lashes *before* you put on mascara. Curling lashes after you apply mascara causes lashes to break.

Tweezers. Choose good tweezers with a lot of spring back and a slanted edge to pluck out excess eyebrow hair and to remove wild hairs from the face.

Scissors. Small, straightedged scissors are used to trim long or wild eyebrow hairs.

The Essential Brushes

There are two things that a woman should not skimp on: cotton sheets and quality makeup brushes. The market offers brushes made from the hairs of sable and blue squirrel and from nylon. If you can afford to, invest in several sable brushes. They have shape memory, no matter what you do to them. Be careful with sable brushes, because color goes exactly where you put it. If you want a sheerer, broad wash of color, the squirrel brush has a lighter touch.

Brushes are the softest, least harmful way to transfer cosmetics to the face. They are used to line the eyes, fill in the lip line, fluff on eye shadow and blusher, smudge harsh lines, and for finishing with powder. Small brushes with shorter, stiffer bristles can be used to train the eyebrows, apply mascara, and remove the excess.

Eyebrow Brush. Use this brush to train your eyebrows by first brushing them upward and then smoothing them back toward the ear.

Powder Brush. The largest brush in your collection fluffs finishing powder onto your face, softens foundation, or blends blusher.

Blusher Brush. Fluffy blusher brushes cut on an angle fit comfortably over the cheekbone. Brushes in blush compacts are too small and pick up too much color.

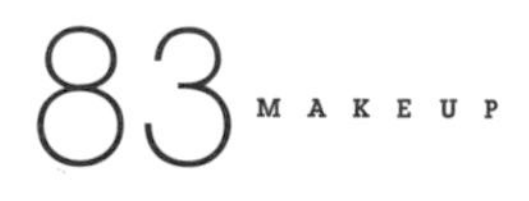

Beauty Tip 02:
If you don't want a lined look but need definition and thickness near the base of the lashes, wet an eye shadow (black, brown, taupe) and use Paula Dorf's brush to push the color into the lashes from beneath. This takes some practice, but the look is natural.

Fantail Brush (optional). I've always loved this brush for easing on just the right amount of blusher, because it fits right over the cheekbone.

Eyeliner Brush. Use this narrow, domed brush to line the eyes with eye-shadow powder or to smudge the line laid down by eyeliner pencils. If your looking for a sharper line, try the Trish McEvoy No. 11 brush. It's ⅜ inches wide and imparts a precise line very close to the base of the lashes. Or try Paula Dorf's tiny nylon brush—its slight curve follows the lash line on the inner side of the lid.

Eye-Shadow Brushes. You will probably want two: a 1-inch soft, fluffy brush to broadcast a sheer wash of color over the whole lid; and a small, soft slanted brush to fit comfortably into the crease under the socket bone for applying contour color.

Spoolie. Looking like a fresh mascara brush with a series of stiff, short bristles arranged horizontally along a central core, the spoolie removes excess mascara.

Lipstick Brush. If you like to line your lips, a brush is an excellent way to fill in lip color without disturbing the precise line of your lip pencil.

Care of Tools

All of these nifty tools and brushes are geared for your face, lips, and around your eyes, where the skin is the thinnest and most tender on your body. One of the most important things you can do for the life, health, and welfare of your skin is to keep your tools clean. Wash your brushes, puffs, and sponges at least once a week. You can use a mild dish liquid, baby shampoo, or simply brush them across your facial soap under tepid running water; then rinse them until you see the water run clean. It isn't necessary to purchase special brush cleaners. They tend to be too strong and can do more damage than good. Never soak your brushes, because water will loosen the glue that holds the bristles to the handle..

The best time to clean your brushes is during your private time, let's say a Saturday or Sunday night, when you turn your bathroom into a private spa. Light some candles, tuck your hair under a shower cap, slather a delicious

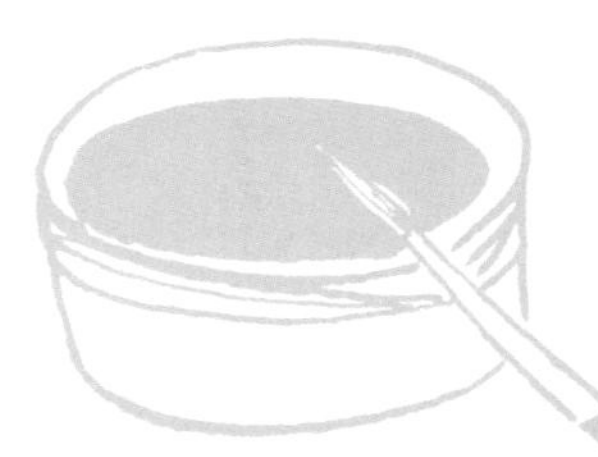

mask or treatment onto your clean face, and settle in to a bath of bubbles, soothing salts, or fragrant oil. When you get out of the tub and towel off, you can wash your brushes and let them dry in the air (stand them up in a tumbler on your vanity or sink). They'll be fresh and waiting for another week's worth of use come Monday morning.

STEP-BY-STEP WITH MAKEUP ESSENTIALS

The time is at hand to choose and apply cosmetics to your face. There is nothing mysterious or daunting about a few pots of foundation, blush, eye shadow, and lipstick. Consider them your crayons and imagine yourself a child again, painting with wild abandon. You can use as many, or as few, of these decorative colors as you'd like. There is no right or wrong way, just *your* way. However, there are some neat tricks that will make putting on makeup simple and fun. And if you don't like what you've done, you can always wash it off.

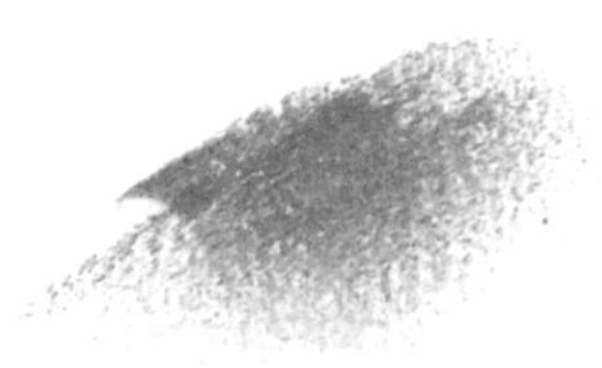

Light some candles, tuck your hair under a shower cap, slather a delicious mask or treatment onto your clean face, and settle in to a bath of bubbles, soothing salts, or fragrant oil.

Step One: Moisturizer

Before you even think of applying foundation to your face, you must prime the canvas. Moisturizer acts as a sealant to keep the skin's natural moisture from evaporating through the pores. Think of your moisturizer as an invisible layer, like cellophane, protecting your skin from environmental insult. Make sure that your moisturizer has at least SPF 15, and use it under your foundation or on your bare face every single day of the year.

Your choice of moisturizer has to do with personal taste. Choose from liquids or creams; oil or no oil; light or heavy. Visit a cosmetic counter and tell the beauty advisor that you are in the market for a new moisturizer. She can recommend something for you according to your skin type. Then ask for samples. Go to a few counters and pick up samples from several brands. Use each sample for two to three days. In that amount of time, you will know if your skin breaks out or if the product clogs your pores. You will also be able

Beauty Tip 03:
When buying concealer, choose a color one shade lighter than your natural skin tone. To neutralize dark circles or redness caused by broken capillaries or a red undertone in the skin, find a concealer that has more yellow in it.

to judge if you like the way the moisturizer feels, smells, and lies on your skin and under your foundation. Then go back and buy the one you like the best.

Step One-and-a-Half: Eye Cream

In the recent past, more and more professional makeup artists have been advising the use of eye cream under your concealer. This is an option. The skin around your eyes is delicate. Very few oil glands hang out there and any emollient has to be put *on* the skin. Eye creams may seem to be an unnecessary expense, but if you experience dryness or itchiness around the eyes, try using a little bit of cream under your foundation to keep the area soft. Again, ask for samples. Try some; you might like it. If not, don't buy it.

All eye creams from topflight cosmetic companies are ophthalmologically and dermatologically tested, and that fact should be marked on the package in plain sight. If you don't find that notation, don't buy the product. And if, while you are sampling an eye cream, it causes your eyes to water, gives you a rash, or makes your eyes itch, discontinue its use immediately.

If you decide to use an eye cream, pat it on right under your eye, from the outside corner to about the center of your iris, using your ring finger. It's best to not put eye cream close to your nose or to the tear ducts, in the inward corner of the eye. Also, avoid covering the eye cream (which will absorb into your skin in about five minutes) with moisturizer. It isn't necessary and will make it doubly hard for your foundation to stay in place.

Step Two: Concealer

When Max Factor marketed Erase, a concealer in a lipstick tube that swirled up conveniently, women used it everywhere—under their eyes to block out dark circles, over their lipstick (especially in the early 1960s) to create new colors, and in facial creases and lines in an attempt to minimize them. It was thought that concealer with foundation over it could work miracles. And for a while it did. But times have changed and heavy, waxy concealers under foundation are yesterday's news, as is a heavy, masklike foundation.

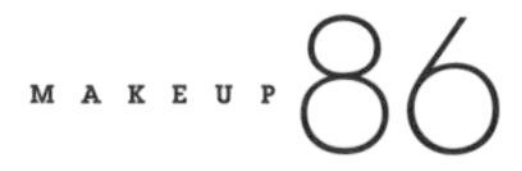

If you watch a professional makeup artist, you'll see that both concealer and foundation are employed with a very light hand, and only in so-called problem areas: to block out dark circles, to obscure blemishes, and to highlight certain areas of the face on top of, not under, foundation. The whole idea is to let the skin shine through. A nice thought for someone who is a dewy 30-year-old, but what about teenaged girls with acne or older women with broken capillaries, sun damage, and those proverbial dark circles? Wearing concealer, then, becomes a choice. Whether you put it on under your foundation as a camouflage or over it to correct imperfections is entirely up to you.

Cream Formula. The heaviest of the concealers on the market comes in a stick form, like Erase, or in a pot, like the one from Stila. This is maximum coverage for minimizing under-eye circles, hiding blemishes, and camouflaging skin imperfections. You can use this type of concealer with a brush, much like your domed eye-shadow brush, for pinpoint accuracy of application. Use your sponge wedge to blend and soften. Be careful when working under your eyes: Too much concealer directly under the eye will achieve a reverse raccoon-eye look. Creams also tend to be greasy and to collect in fine lines, so use it sparingly and blend it in slightly by tapping with your ring finger or with a soft, clean sponge.

Tube. The texture of concealer from a tube is thinner and creamier than stick concealer and works up like foundation. You can find this product in oil-free formulas. Use it with a small, domed brush for directed coverage and blend with the pointed end of a sponge wedge.

Liquid with Sponge Applicator. This type of concealer is packaged the same way as lip gloss and mascara are, that is, in a convenient plastic tube with an applicator. You can control the amount of concealer you use because this formula is as sheer as some foundations. In fact, you can use it to even out your skin tone and forgo foundation entirely. The wand style is highly portable, so you can carry it in your makeup kit or purse for quick touch-ups during the day.

Beauty Tip 04: Use your sheerest concealer as a substitute for eye-shadow base.

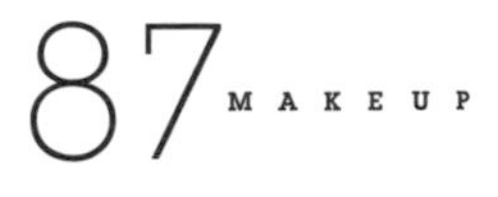

What Kind of Coverage Do I Need?

- **Light.** A sheer foundation base with a dewy finish will even out color without covering up skin tone or freckles.
- **Medium.** For most skin types, this is a good program to follow. Medium coverage will address the redness in your skin and neutralize it. Don't expect medium coverage to mask sun spots or dark circles.
- **Heavy.** You run the risk of emphasizing fine lines and wrinkles with heavier coverage, but a foundation with a smooth, matte finish will hide dominant flaws such as acne scars, rosacea, and sun spots.

Pencil Stick. Concealer in skinny or chubby pencil form puts the product where you want it with pinpoint accuracy and is good for masking pesky pimples or correcting smeared makeup around the eyes or lip line.

Step Three: Foundation

If you've never used foundation, you might ask yourself: "Why should I? I would feel as if I were wearing a mask." Perhaps, in the relative dark ages of makeup application, you would have. There have been periods when women applied foundation thickly, as if they wanted to hide more than their skin. In the 1950s, the trend was to overcompensate for yellow skin undertones. So-called neutral beiges included a lot of pink. So when it was applied to the face, the line of demarcation between where foundation stopped and natural skin began was obvious. Makeup for women of color in the 1950s was not always successful because very few companies took into consideration that the titanium dioxide in foundation turned ashy on darker skins.

Today, the trend in foundation is to wear a color as close to your own skin tone as possible and to use as little as possible for coverage—just enough to augment natural skin tone, to even out imperfections, or to give skin a finished appearance under artificial lighting. Modern foundations are lightweight, supersheer, and buildable; you can put on as little or as much as you want for a finished look. They also come in full color ranges, from the lightest, most ivory hue to the darkest mahogany. Treatment makeup is also available; foundation can be purchased with any number of skin-enhancing additives.

SPF (Sun Protection Factor). If you don't want to put it on separately, or if your moisturizer doesn't already have an SPF, make sure your face is protected by choosing a foundation with at least SPF 15 in it.

AHA/BHA. American women tend to overuse these exfoliating products. Some foundations advertise that they contain these fruit acids, which I don't understand. Why would you want exfoliators in a foundation that should last all day? If you use an AHA or BHA at all, it's best do it at night while your skin rests and repairs. AHA in foundation is overkill that can cause dryness, irritation, and breakouts.

Antioxidants. Vitamin C, vitamin E, and ceremides in a foundation could be a prescription for more skin problems. They do protect your skin from environmental pollution and free radicals, but if you break out, stop using the foundation. Ceremides are an invention of the cosmetic industry, a form of "cosmeceutical," often a delivery system of certain serums onto the skin's surface and then sub-dermally.

Oil-Absorbing Products. Some foundations use kaolin and talc in an effort to control excess oil and to keep the foundation matte. Eventually, with the natural buildup of dirt and grime that occurs during the day, you could look like you're wearing a mask.

Types of Foundation

Tinted Moisturizer. Light and sheer, tinted moisturizers are considered sport makeups. They usually have an SPF in them and give you all the benefits of a moisturizer, protecting your skin as they color it ever so slightly. You can expect a glow from the sport tint, but no appreciable coverage. If you have young, relatively unblemished skin, tinted moisturizers are an excellent introduction to wearing foundation base on your face. *The finished effect: a natural glow.*

Sheer Liquid Foundation. Most large cosmetic companies make a sheer base in a large color range. Sheer means sheer. Don't expect allover coverage; this product will just even out skin tone. Sheers also dry very quickly, so you have to learn to work fast, blending one area at a time. Start by dotting a bit on your forehead, blending outward from the center with either clean fingers or a soft, clean sponge. Move next to your cheeks, then your chin. Use the excess on your sponge to get your nose and any spots you've missed. *The finished effect: a silky, smooth face.*

Beauty Tip 05:
Try this trick. To finish your foundation, form your sponge into a soft cone. Turn it on your face, gently going counterclockwise, from area to area. Your foundation will have a more stippled, natural look, and the sponge will remove excess foundation from your pores. This little trick also sets your foundation and eliminates the need for powder.

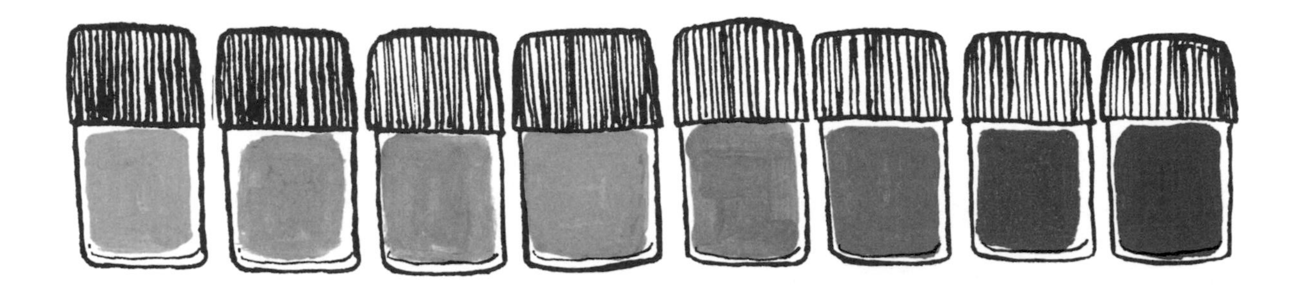

Selecting the Right Foundation Color

When choosing the color of your foundation, remember to always match your skin exactly. And if you can't find a foundation that is as close to an exact match as possible in existing color lines, have one custom blended. The cost is not prohibitive. The goal here is for foundation to disappear on your face, to let your own natural skin tone show through. Here are some pointers:

- **For Caucasian women:**
  If you look good in paper-white clothes, you probably have a cool complexion. Look for cooler, ivory shades.
  If you look better in an off-white, cream, or beige, you've got a warm complexion. Look for warmer tones of beige.

- **For women of color:** Determine the undertone of your skin—Hispanic, Asian, or African American skin can have either a red or yellow undertone.

Emulsion Liquid Foundation. These are medium-weight liquids, a combination of oil and water. Shake the bottle well before use. These foundations may be enriched with treatment elements such as vitamin E or ceremides, which means your skin gets moisturized as you cover it. This is an especially good foundation for normal-to-dry skin and for aging skin, particularly if it has at least SPF 15 in it. It is a humectant and feels moist on your face. You can get very good coverage with just a little bit, blended with your fingers or a soft sponge. *The finished effect: satiny, dewy skin.*

Oil-Free Liquid Foundation. Sensitive skin that pumps out an excess of sebum appreciates this kind of foundation. It glides on easily because silicates have been used instead of oils. Oil-free foundations provide greater coverage over minor eruptions and acne scars, but you could end up with a makeup mask if you use a heavy hand. Also, these foundations take a little getting used to because they feel fairly tacky on the skin until they dry. *The finished effect: medium coverage with a demi-matte surface.*

Water-Based, Oil-Free Foundation. Don't like a base with oil? Have problems cleaning your face? This is a foundation for you. You can get sheer-to-medium coverage with this type of base, especially if you apply it with a sponge. It washes off quickly with water. *The finished effect: slightly matte, slightly moist.*

Cream Foundation. Buy this base in a pot and apply it with your fingers. Usually high in oil content, this foundation gives the heaviest coverage and is geared to aging and older skins. A little bit goes a long way, especially when you warm it with the heat of your fingers before you smooth it on. The finish is luxurious and slightly humectant. Cream foundation also gives you a gorgeous finish for special occasion nights. *The finished effect: full coverage with a satiny finish.*

Cream-to-Powder Compact. This highly portable base is practical if you're away from home all day and need a mid-afternoon touchup. Thick in texture, this makeup is used with a sponge, goes on like a cream, and dries to a slightly matte finish. But beware, you can make mistakes with this foundation, because it is tempting to put on a lot. Cream-to-powders are good for slightly oily skin or to achieve a smooth, velvety appearance. Since they dry down to a matte, finishing powder is not necessary. *The finished effect: even texture with a demi-matte finish.*

Swivel-Stick Foundation. Combining both concealer and foundation in a swivel-up tube, these look like massive lipsticks. They are very portable and convenient but the texture is thick and dense. The heavier you use it, the more coverage you get. These are excellent for black and white photography (which is why cosmetic genius Max Factor developed the PanStick in the first place), but they look anything but natural. *The finished effect: total opaque coverage.*

Long-Wearing Foundation. Foundation, like lipstick, is available in long-wear formulas that require special cleansers to remove. This foundation is very convenient if you are gone all day and aren't able to retouch your makeup. However, on older skin, it is drying and tends to look heavy and masklike. *The finished effect: long-wearing full coverage.*

Water Canvas Foundation. Cool to the touch, this high-tech makeup looks like a cream, feels like a gel, but breaks down into a liquid the moment a sponge touches its surface. It leaves a sheer matte finish and is very good for younger skin; however, it tends to look flaky, dry, and powdery on older skin. Also, if you do not shut the compact tightly, it can dry out. *The finished effect: a sheer matte.*

Light-Refracting Foundation. The latest wrinkle (no pun intended) in foundation has been the addition of light-refracting ingredients (mica or fish scales), which give older skin the appearance of youth and dewiness. If your skin has started to lose its ability to slough off dead skin cells quickly and is losing elasticity and moisture, this new foundation will refract light and make your skin appear to glow from the outside. *The finished effect: a sheer, youthful glow.*

- Shop with a face clear of cosmetics.
- At the cosmetic counter, try on foundation by painting a stripe at your jawline, as close to your neck as possible (you have less sun damage there). If you cannot see the foundation, if it disappears into your natural skin tone, that's the color you should buy.
- Come to the cosmetic counter with a mirror; go outside or close to a window and look at the stripes of foundation on your face in natural light.
- Take advantage of the cosmetic company's sampling policy. Go home with samples of the foundation you've chosen; wear it for a few days to see whether you break out and whether it feels good and wears well. If so, and you like it: Buy it.

Facing Up to Face Powder

- Loose powder smooths and polishes, lends finish to, and sets foundation.
- Choose a translucent powder, one that is very sheer and has almost no color in it for a basic finish.
- Carry a pressed powder in the same shade as your loose powder for touch-ups during the day.
- For a sheer look, use a brush-on pressed powder instead of a puff.
- Loose powder doubles as an eye shadow base or a matte finish for your lipstick.
- Loose powders with glitter particles or metallics lend a festive evening look to makeup. Try fluffing glitter powders on your shoulders, collarbone, and décolletage.

Step Four: Face Powder

Face powder, like red lipstick, comes in and out of vogue constantly. A lovely dusting of translucent powder over your foundation fixes your makeup and gives it a smooth, demi-matte finish. With cream-to-powder foundations or mattes, you really don't need it. But if your makeup tends to run or disappear by noon, a thin layer of powder, fluffed on lightly with a large, soft brush, ensures some longevity. It smoothes the skin and adds polish to any makeup. However, if you're using one of the light-refracting foundations where the idea is to appear as moist, young, and dewy as possible, face powder is not appropriate.

So far, you've been preparing your face to accept its accessories—the jewels of the face: eye makeup, lipstick, and blusher. With moisturizer, concealer, foundation, and loose powder, you've covered blemishes, evened out texture and tone, and given your face its perfect finish. Now it's time to play with color.

There is some disagreement over what should come next—blusher or eye makeup. My thought is: Do your eyes and your mouth first, then put on blush. Here's why. Eye makeup and lipstick attract the eye. They add focus to a face. In fashion, the rule of thumb has always been either strong eyes and light lips or strong lips and light eyes. This is what makeup designers have been saying for years. However, if you are *not* aiming for a high-fashion look, then your lips and eyes should achieve some sort of balance. Do what you want. It's your face, and your makeup is a matter of your taste.

Do you like a lot of mascara? Then by all means, stroke it on. Red lips and dark eyeliner for that retro 1950s look? Why not, if it's you? If you are not sure, then the following instructions for fairly neutral makeup are a good place to start. Then, once you see how vivid your lips are and how dark your eye makeup is, add blusher as the finishing touch.

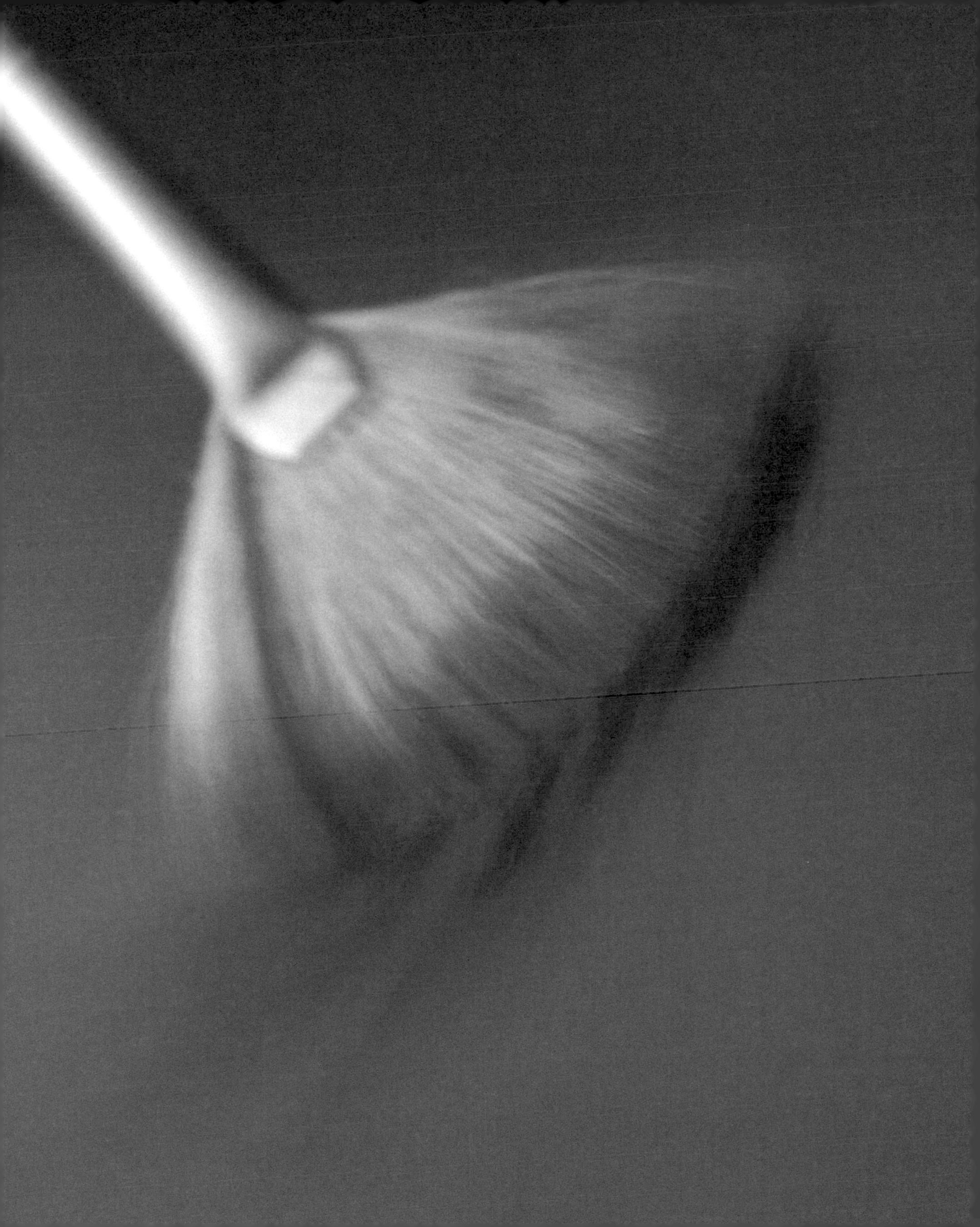

Beauty Tip 06:

When you apply loose powder, use a powder brush. Avoid powder puffs. They do not remove the excess; they smoosh it in.

Step Five: Eyebrow Treatment

The eyebrow is the single most important feature on your face. It can make or break your makeup. Eyebrows move independent of your consciousness. They are a reflection of what you're really feeling. They can knit up in concern and dismay. They arch in surprise and irony. They can convey meaning just by their shape and texture alone.

Unkempt brows do you a disservice. If they are too thick or extend across the bridge of your nose, people might see you as angry. If they are too thin, you may appear an affected snob. Properly tweezed and trained eyebrows can mean the difference between looking like a little girl and looking like a grown-up woman. Brows are the one feature of your face that you can change without plastic surgery.

If you've never had your eyebrows done and they look wild and unkempt, the ideal approach is to have them tweezed or waxed professionally. Your hairdresser will probably be able to recommend a good makeup artist or facialist who knows what she is doing. But if the cost is prohibitive, then you should learn to do your brows yourself.

Brow Shaping by the Numbers

1. Provide yourself with good light, either at your bathroom mirror or seated at a table near a bright window.
2. Brush your eyebrows up first and then toward your ear to see if you have long, wild hairs that can be trimmed with your small straight-edged scissors.
3. To determine the arch, lower your chin toward your chest, forcing your eyebrows up as far as they will go. With your fingers, determine the highest point in the brow before it tapers downward toward your ear. This is the arch.
4. Looking straight into the mirror, note that the apex of your eyebrow is directly over the part of your iris nearest the side of your face.

⑤ Your eyebrows should start directly over the inside corner of your eye and end slightly past the outside corner. To find the precise starting and stopping points, you can use a straight edge or a pencil.

- To find where your eyebrows should begin, lay your pencil, orange stick (see page 160), or small ruler perpendicularly from your mouth, alongside your nose and past your brow. Where the brow and pencil intersect is where the brow should begin. Any hairs that march over toward the center of your nose past the straight edge should be removed.
- To find where your brow should end, take your straight edge and, starting from the center of your chin, lay it in a diagonal line from the chin past the outside corner of your eye. Where the pencil or ruler intersects with the brow is where it should taper to an end.

⑥ Now that you know its placement, it's time to sketch your ideal brow. You want to take out only those hairs that obscure your natural arch. You can rehearse by using a combination of eyebrow pencil and white eyeliner pencil. Sketch your ideal eyebrow with the pencil or with a small, slanted-edged brush and brown eye shadow. Block out the hairs you don't want with white liner pencil or a concealer pencil. These are the hairs you will tweeze away.

⑦ Tweezing hurts, so you may want to deaden the area before you tweeze by pressing an ice cube on it for about 15 seconds. When you are finished, the skin may be red and sore. A cotton ball dipped in witch hazel will cool the area and prevent swelling.

⑧ If your eyebrows are light (blondes often have almost invisible hairs) or sparse, you can fill in the blanks with a soft shade of brown, charcoal gray, or taupe using a slanted-edged brush. You can fix the look with a careful application of transparent, colorless mascara or a brow-fix product.

Beauty Tip 07:

After you've finished coloring in your brows with either pencil or the brush/shadow method, take your brow-fix product, which has an applicator that looks like a mascara brush, and, using the pointed end instead of the side, retrace the shape of your brow, moving the color around until you like it. Take a tissue and blot off the excess.

Step Six: Eyeliner, Eye Shadow, and Mascara

The old poetic cliché that the eyes are the windows of the soul is right. Your eyes talk when your lips don't, and often they give you away. Have a conversation with someone who asks too many personal questions, and while your lips may be smiling politely, your eyes are probably blank and expressionless or even focused somewhere other than on the offending person. If you are angry, perhaps your eyes change color. And if you're touched by a sentimental memory, maybe your eyes tear up unexpectedly. You owe it to your eyes to make them as expressive and lovely as possible, emphasizing their positive aspects—long lashes, a graceful shape, extraordinary color or placement—with color, liner, and mascara.

Lining Your Eyes. Depending upon what kind of eyeliner you like—precise or smudged—you can line your eyes with an eyeliner pencil, a tiny domed brush and eye shadow powder, or liquid liner. The latter will give you a very precise line, but it tends to look harsh, takes a lot of practice, and occasionally, leaves a mirror print on the upper part of your eyelid if you didn't let it dry. Unless you buy a waterproof product, liquid liner can dissolve with your tears.

With eye pencil, brush, and powder, or liquid liner get the line as close to your lashes as possible, almost as if you wanted to color the root of the lash, not the skin around it. This will help any sparse lashes appear thicker at the root, and naturally thick lashes will look outrageously luxurious.

My favorite way to line the eyes is with brush and powder. Take your fine, small brush and stroke it gently across a dark shade of eye-shadow powder—charcoal, dark brown, taupe, or black; the amount you use will depend on how dramatic a look you want. Determine how much powder you have on your brush by using your hand as your tester palette. When you've gotten the desired effect on your hand, press the brush as close to your lash line as possible on your upper lid. Here is where the Trish McEvoy No. 11 brush can come in handy. Use the dip-and-press method; avoid dragging the brush along the lash line. The tapered edged of this brush is so precise that you can even line your eyes in minute sections, getting very close to your natural lashes to press in a fine line of color.

If you're using a pencil, sharpen it first, then dull the edge a bit with the warmth of your palm and draw gently with tiny, feathery strokes. It is not necessary to put liner on in one long, unbroken line. Tiny, intersecting strokes accomplish the same effect and are kinder to the delicate skin around the eye.

It is not necessary to line under your lower lashes, but if you do, try to keep the two lines—upper and lower—from intersecting, because that will tend to make the eye look smaller. To soften your line, you can use a cotton swab, a small sponge applicator, or a clean lipstick brush.

Eye Shadow. Remember the "Face Game" exercise earlier in this chapter? Close your eyes once again and feel the eyelid as it extends from the upper lash line to the area right under your occipital bone, or eye socket. For a sheer wash of color, use the brush that most resembles a watercolor brush. For simple makeup, stick to neutrals to even out your lid color—a soft buff, beige, ecru, taupe, lavender, or celadon. Cover the entire lid area, after testing the amount of shadow you've put on your brush using the back of your hand.

If you've lined your eyes and brushed a single color on your lids, the next step may be to simply apply mascara to your lashes and forget about any fancy shading. But if you'd like to set off your eyelid, contouring is fairly simple if you have the right brush. You can use a dome-top eye-shadow brush, which has bristles a little less flexible than those of the brush you've used for your color wash. Feel how the brush fits comfortably in the recessed area beneath your occipital bone, up close and personal with your eye socket. Starting at the outside edge of your eye and working inward, stroke on a slightly darker color than the one you used on your lid.

Be sure to blend any color you put around your eyes, letting the colors flow into each other. There should be no line of demarcation, just a seamless transition from one color to the next. You can also brush on a much lighter color (even lighter than the shade you've used on your eyelid) to highlight the area right under the arch of your eyebrow.

Beauty Tip 08:

Glitter shadows may be very pretty and appealing in the pot, but on your eyes, they can age you if the skin around your eyes is dry or has developed fine lines. Use them sparingly with a very light hand.

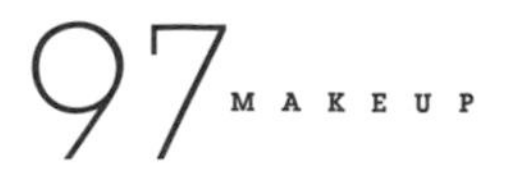

Beauty Tip 09:
Try using your blusher as the contour color for your eye makeup. The pink, coral, or rose will lift the eye and make it sparkle.

For evening, you may want to consider a shimmer shadow for a festive touch. Avoid using a paper-white highlighter; that can look theatrical and dated. Choose a very pale shade of lemon, pink, off-white, cream, or pearl, and place it directly under the eyebrow, tracing the arch. Highlighter shadow should be so sheer that it is just a whisper, a hint of color. Do not extend the highlighter past the outside of the brow. Be sure to blend well so that the margin of the color disappears.

Eye Makeup Options

- **Creamy pencil.** Pencils contain wax, petroleum, or silicates and leave a strong, defining line.
- **Powder and brush.** Use eye shadow and a small domed brush for a more muted eyeliner. Smudge it for a soft effect.
- **Eye shadow powder.** This comes in a compact or a small pot and is applied with a brush; it can be used wet for intensity and drama.
- **Eye-shadow stick.** Popularized in the 1950s, the eye crayon was very greasy and tended to run when it warmed up or to lodge itself in the creases of the eyelid. Newer formulas with silicates dry down to a powdery finish.
- **Cream-to-powder eye shadow.** This comes in a mascara-like rod with a sponge applicator, or in a tube. You have about a 30-second window to manipulate it on your eyelids; stroke it on for obvious color, or thin to a light color wash with your finger.
- **Chubby crayon.** This usually has a cream-to-powder texture; it can be stroked on the lid for shadow or used as a halo of liner around the eye. Some have shimmer.
- **Liquid eyeliner.** Liquid liner requires some practice in the application; it gives a very precise line, but can look harsh if applied too thickly.

Beauty Tip 10:
If time is a factor, mascara and a vibrant red lipstick alone can look dramatic and fabulous.

Mascara. Think of the final swish of mascara as a finishing touch—like clipping on your earrings or dabbing scent on your pulse points. Mascara is the final step to a complete eye makeup.

Modern mascara comes in a wand format; a thin rod topped with a brush is inserted into a plastic or metallic tube that holds the formula. Mascara formulas vary depending upon what effect they provide.

- **Thickening** formula coats each lash; some formulas "swell" on the lash to make them look thicker.
- **Lengthening** formula may contain polymer fibers that adhere to the tips of your lashes to make them appear longer. These fibers can be irritating and make your eyes tear, or they can cause the lashes to break if the mascara is inexpensive and drying.
- **Conditioning** formula will contain vitamin E to help your lashes look silky and luxuriant.
- **Waterproof** formula is difficult to get off; you may need a special solvent or mascara remover. Although waterproofs are great for sports, continuous use could cause your lashes to break.

When you shop for a mascara, also consider the brush. The thicker the brush, the more bristles it has and the more mascara it can carry to your lashes. For sparse lashes, try a smaller brush. Avoid brushes that bring a surfeit of mascara, which can glob and smear.

Apply your mascara by starting at the root of the lashes, following the curve of the lashes, upward and outward. Don't let your mascara collect at the tips. Brushing mascara on the lower lashes is a matter of choice and is a trend that comes and goes. I know women who would feel naked without their bottom lashes coated, but you have to be careful. To get a precise application that will not end up as a dark smudge under your eyes, turn your mascara wand perpendicular to your lash line, and paint only a few lashes at the outside corner; paint each lash singly with the tip of the wand.

If you like your lashes to look spiky, as if each one had been coated separately, look for mascara applicators that are simply a series of grooves cut all

Rule of Thumb:

Choose a color most like your natural hair color for eye contouring. Copper works well with auburn or red hair; charcoal gray or off-black work with dark hair; brown, with chestnut or brunette hair; and taupe and darker tan work well with blonde hair.

Beauty Tip 11:

If you can't put on mascara without getting a lot on the skin below your eye, try bending the tip to an angle, like a dentist's mirror, to give you more control.

Beauty Tip 12:

Be sure to curl your eyelashes *before* you apply mascara. If you use your curler while your lashes are wet or after the mascara is dry, you can cause major breakage. To get the best curl out of your lashes, use a blow dryer on your curler for about 10 seconds to heat it up. It's like using a curling iron on your hair.

the way around the rod (Clinique and Chanel wands offer this method of application), which trap the lashes and coat them. This type of applicator works very well if your lashes are thin and short. To remove excess mascara, use either an eyebrow brush or a spoolie, which looks like an unused mascara brush. You can use this excess mascara to darken your brows.

Step Seven: Lipstick

Lipstick is probably the first thing you borrowed from your mother's dresser when you were a little girl playing dress up. And when you were 13, it marked your passage into puberty. Now that you're grown, it's probably what you stuff in your pocket or evening bag when you leave the house. You'd forget your house keys and your checkbook. But your lipstick? Never!

I have to confess, I love lipstick. In my medicine chest (where you couldn't find an aspirin if your life depended on it), I must have at least 25 to 30 lipsticks at any given time, most of them varying shades of red: brown-red, blue-red, red-red, sheer red, matte red, clear red. To me, lipstick is a ritual in a tube, one that I probably learned from my mother. There is something so tactile, so sexy, about the feel of a metal tube in the hand, the slight muffled pop when you remove the cap, the feeling of anticipation and expectation as you twist the tube to swivel up the color. Then you put it on and voila! Your face has brightened; your eye color pops; and even if you're only wearing lipstick, somehow you feel . . . dressed.

Whether I am buying a lipstick or just window shopping, I feel a magical lift when I see all those brilliant colors, just waiting for me to choose.

Not all women think that they can wear lipstick, let alone red lipstick. It's just a matter of matching your own taste with what is on the market. Lipsticks are all basically the same, whether they are creamy, matte, sheer, or glossy. They are made of wax, oil, pigment, and fragrance, supplied in varying proportions and they are a low-cost, high-profit item. The industry's rule of thumb is for every 25¢ worth of ingredients, the cosmetic company adds $10. So if you buy a $22.50 lipstick, you can bet that there is less than $1.50 worth of materials in it.

Beauty Tip 13:
If toward the end of the day, your makeup has suddenly disappeared, try reapplying your lipstick, and watch how the color takes away sallowness and fatigue.

If you hate wearing lipstick, consider what you don't like about it. It's too goopy. It gets on your teeth. Your mouth stands out. You're sure everybody is looking at you. You feel like a fallen woman. Some of these attitudes probably date back to your mother's teaching, and maybe you should reconsider. You are ripe for experimentation and play. Ease into wearing lipstick by trying something fairly low-key, like a sheer gloss. If you absolutely do not like color but have been protecting your lips with some other kind of lip treatment, then a clear or delicately tinted gloss would work for you, since you're used to having something on your lips. From there, you can progress to other forms of lip color.

Lip Gloss. The sheerest, most emollient form of lip color, gloss comes in either a wand, like mascara, with a brush or sponge-tip applicator or in a pot. The texture is slippery like Vaseline, with color ranges from no pigment (clear gloss) to natural tones such as blush pink, rose, and peach, to colored glosses that look dark in the pot but go on like a sheer tint. Gloss can make you look sporty or girlish and is fine for the minimalist, no-makeup look. *Problem: Lip gloss is a high-maintenance item that requires constant reapplication.*

Lip Lacquer. A fairly recent industrial-strength lip gloss, lacquer also comes with sponge or brush applicator or in a pot. Lacquer has intense pigment with a high degree of shine. On the lip, it looks like stained glass—a lot of color but not opaque. High maintenance and very flashy, lacquer will deposit on anything from cups and silverware to your teeth if you're not careful. *Problem: Lacquer runs and feathers. If you have teensy vertical lines around your mouth, it would be best to avoid using it.*

Sheer Formula. Although this type is available in a classic swivel-up tube, it acts like a gloss. It has more emollient than pigment, which gives it a tinted, transparent appearance on the lips. A sheer can slick on like a classic gloss, or you can build it up for more color. *Problem: Like gloss, sheer requires constant tending and reapplication.*

Cream Formula. Of the tube-type lipstick, this is the most humectant. The newer cream formulas are jazzed up with vitamin E,

Beauty Tip 14: When you want a more natural-appearing lip but you'd like to wear color that won't eat off, try covering your entire lip with a pencil, one shade darker than your natural lip tone, softening it with your finger, and then slicking on some transparent gloss.

ceremides, and SPF so they condition and protect as they color. Cream formula has a definite weight on your lips but tends to feel the best when you first put it on. The latest formulas are made with silicates rather than oils and tend not to wander. *Problem: Cream formula can feel heavy and leaves lip prints if you don't blot it.*

Matte Formula. If you're looking for a nonshiny lipstick that dries down to a flat finish, one that appears very deep and velvety, then a matte is for you. *Problem: It can be very drying.*

Creamy Matte Formula. Sound contradictory? The latest matte goes on like a cream, smooth and emollient. Because it contains silicates, it will dry to a demi-shiny finish; it won't wander, and it will continue to feel like a cream but certainly won't look like one. In one lipstick, you can have it both ways. *Problem: Because it is pigment rich, it may leave a trace of color on your lips even after you've removed your makeup.*

Nontransfer Formula. This used to be called indelible lipstick. It was difficult to remove and tended to dry the lip. The new kind has a demi-matte surface and is removable with special products designed to lift off all color. *Problem: It still tends to dry the lips.*

Transformer. Usually a black- or white-hued sheer formula, this is designed to lighten or darken your existing lipstick wardrobe. It was developed for women who really love their favorite lipsticks and are reluctant to buy a new lipstick just to follow trends, but who still want to look modern. *Problem: Not too many—these are tools for experimentation.*

Lipstick Pencil. Usually a soft, waxy formulation, this is the most intensely pigmented of all lip products. It is designed to line the lips to prevent feathering, to provide a guideline, or to be applied as a lipstick. Remember that lip pencil may alter the color of your lipstick, making it either darker or lighter. *Problem: Some formulas tend to be very drying.*

Lipstick Brush. Using a lipstick brush can be a tricky proposition. But if you want a neat, exact mouth, a brush is the best way to achieve it. If you've outlined your lips in pencil, simply pass your lip brush over the surface of your lipstick a few times and then paint inside the lines. If you have

an old lipstick brush around, don't throw it out. Wash it carefully and use it to smudge your eyeliner. *Problem: Lipstick brushes require practice for precision.*

Applying Lipstick

Before you even start contemplating your lips, get them into excellent condition. If you bite your lips or if they're chapped, make a lip conditioner part of your everyday regimen, both at night before you go to sleep, and in the morning before you put on your lipstick.

Using your chin as an anchor, rest your pinkie finger to steady your lip pencil (if you choose to line your lips). If you want a precise line, use a freshly sharpened pencil and feathery, little interlocking strokes. Start with your biggest lip first; then you can judge if you have to help the other lip by making it a little larger. In the "Face Game" earlier in this chapter, you found the outside ridge of your lips. Use that as your borderline, either drawing your lip pencil right below the ridge or directly on it.

On your upper lip, define the bow first and then work downward with gentle, light strokes to the corners of your mouth. You can then fill in your lips with lipstick straight from the tube or with a brush.

You lips will shrink as you get older. There are creative ways of making your lips look fuller, short of collagen injections (remember Goldie Hawn's exaggerated lips in *The First Wives' Club?*). If you've played the "Face Game" and felt your lips with your fingers, you already know that your lips are larger than you think they are. Instead of exaggerating your lips and redrawing them completely, à la Joan Crawford, use a lip liner on the outside edge of the lip on the top and on the inside edge on the bottom.

The Myth and Magic of Red Lipstick

I've always believed in the curative powers of a red lipstick. I've seen the judicious application of a cherry red brighten up the worst day; red lipstick has the ability to lift your spirits and change your attitude.

- **Red has the power to draw the eye directly to the lip.**

Rule of Thumb:

If one of your lips is smaller than the other and you'd like to even them out, line the smallest lip along the outside margin of your lip border (but not beyond it). You can also use a slightly lighter lipstick color on the smaller lip to make it look larger or daub a highlighter in the center of the smaller lip.

- **Poets have always referred to lips in terms of shades of red**—*ruby lips, lips as red as cherries,* and so on. Somehow, *medium-brown lips* doesn't seem quite as romantic.
- **Red lips are fraught with Freudian meaning.** They are thought to be the outward manifestation of a woman's labia and, therefore, instruments of sexual promise. If a woman paints her lips red, is she inviting exploration of what is usually hidden?
- **Red lipstick is the first thing a man notices** about a woman and the last thing she leaves behind—on a Champagne flute, a cigarette, a napkin, or a cheek. Red lipstick is her calling card, her territorial imperative, her X-marks-the-spot.

I believe that any woman can wear a red lipstick, if it is the right color red. First you have to identify whether your skin tone is warm or cool. Again, if you look great in paper-white shirts, your skin probably has cooler, pinky tones; a red with some blue in it is just for you. If you prefer creams and off-whites, then you've got some gold or yellow in your skin and should stay in the warm range, reds that have brown or gold in them. Orange-red lipsticks take a lot of courage—they wear you.

For women of color, determine whether your skin's undertone is red or yellow. Women with an amber or golden undertone can wear a true red, a coral-red, or even a blue-red; women with a reddish undertone can wear darker reds that are closer to burgundy or brown.

Another criterion for wearing red lipstick is to choose the ideal intensity. You might not want to dive into an opaque cream the first time out; instead, choose a red tone with training wheels—like a sheer or a gloss. Wear it around all day; notice what people say to you. Establish a baseline comfort level. If you have decided to brave a red lipstick, consult with a makeup artist and give him or her as much information as you can. The artist can help you determine if what you want is just a hint of color or a real statement. And believe me, red lips do make a statement. They are hard to ignore.

Beauty Tip 15:

To avoid getting lipstick on your teeth, do what models do. Form your mouth into an O and insert your forefinger. The excess lipstick that would ordinarily stain your teeth comes off on your finger.

Beauty Tip 16:
If you don't like the shape of your mouth, don't emphasize it; play up your eyes instead.

Step Eight: Blusher

Applying blusher is where women make the biggest mistakes. You can ruin a look by overdoing your cheek color—wearing too much or putting it in the wrong place. There have been makeup trends when the cheeks were the area of focus. In the 1970s and 1980s, extreme contouring was in, especially in some of the high-fashion photos of Helmut Newton and on the 6-foot tall model Verushka. Mostly, however, makeup artists have either left blusher off the face in the 1990s or mixed a little lipstick with Vaseline and stroked it on as an afterthought. In the millennium, pinky cheeks are back.

Modern blush is sheer and natural with colors in the delicately muted pink, rose, and brown tones. If you dip your head down between your knees for a count of 10 and then look at your face in the mirror, you'll see how you look with a natural blush. Is it too red? Too vivid? Too embarrassing? Then apply your blusher accordingly—with a very light touch.

You've already identified where to put your blusher—along the apex of the cheekbone, the area called the apple of your cheek, tapering slightly toward (but not into) your ear. An easy way to find the top of your cheek bone is to lay a pencil along a line that runs diagonally from the center of your ear to the bottom edge of your nose. The pencil will recline directly on your cheekbone.

The most common form of blusher is a pressed power that comes in a pot or compact that may include a tiny brush with soft bristles set close together. Try not to use this brush for your initial application. Full-sized blusher brushes are designed so you can plop them perpendicularly into the blush pot to pick up color with the tips of the bristles. Test how much you've put on your brush on the back of your hand and then stroke it lightly, from the apple of your cheek back toward your ear. If you think you've put on too much, take your velour puff and blend it in. You can always build up the color if you are pale.

Save your blusher until last, and apply it in balance with your lips and your eyes. You may not need very much if either your lips or eyes are to be the focus of your face. Stay away from using blusher on your temples, forehead, or chin. For evening, especially if you're going to be in a low-light or candlelit situation, darken your blusher a shade or two. You might even consider contouring by adding a darker shade to the hollow right under your cheekbone to play up the contrast. For festive occasions, consider slicking the very top of your cheekbone with a highlighter or some glitter.

Blushers are available in these forms:

Powder Blusher. Like eye shadow, powder blusher is applied with a brush. Some powders have been infused with cream and feel silky to the touch. These are the easiest to control and build.

Cream Blusher. Formerly called rouge, this blusher is creamy and slightly oily to the touch. It is applied with the fingers. The newer cream blushers have quick-drying silicates in them for color that which won't sink into your face after a few hours. You've got about 30 seconds of playtime to manipulate, thin out, and arrange it before it starts to dry.

Stick Blusher. A fairly new product, the swivel-up blusher looks like an oversized lipstick. Direct the blusher precisely where you want it and blend easily.

Gel Blusher. This comes in a tube or pot and tends to take a lot of practice. It's not good for older skin because the alcohol in it can be very drying.

Tint. Usually a liquid (like BeneFit's BeneTint); the application takes some practice. You could look like Betty Boop if you're not careful.

Bronzer. Brownish in hue, this gives your face a warm, healthy appearance. To look sun kissed, you can use it for blusher, or brush it over the entire surface of your face, neck, and chest. It's also good for touch-ups when your tan or fake tanner is fading.

WHAT MAKEUP COLORS SHOULD I USE?

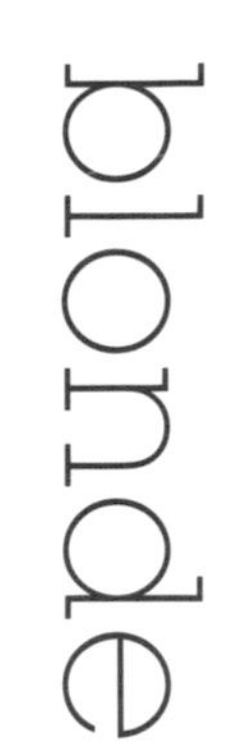

BLONDE: If your skin, lashes, and brows are very pale, define them. You are very lucky. You can look demurely sweet or va-va-va-voom just by changing your lipstick. For a natural look, try a pink or brownish-rose gloss; for nighttime flirtation, definitely a red lipstick. If you're a light blonde—platinum, baby blonde, or ash—you can wear a clear red or a blue-red. If you look like a tawny California blonde with gold tints in your hair and skin, then wear a light dusting of peach-brown blusher and a brown-red lipstick. If your skin tends to pink undertones, emphasize it with pink or fuchsia lipstick.

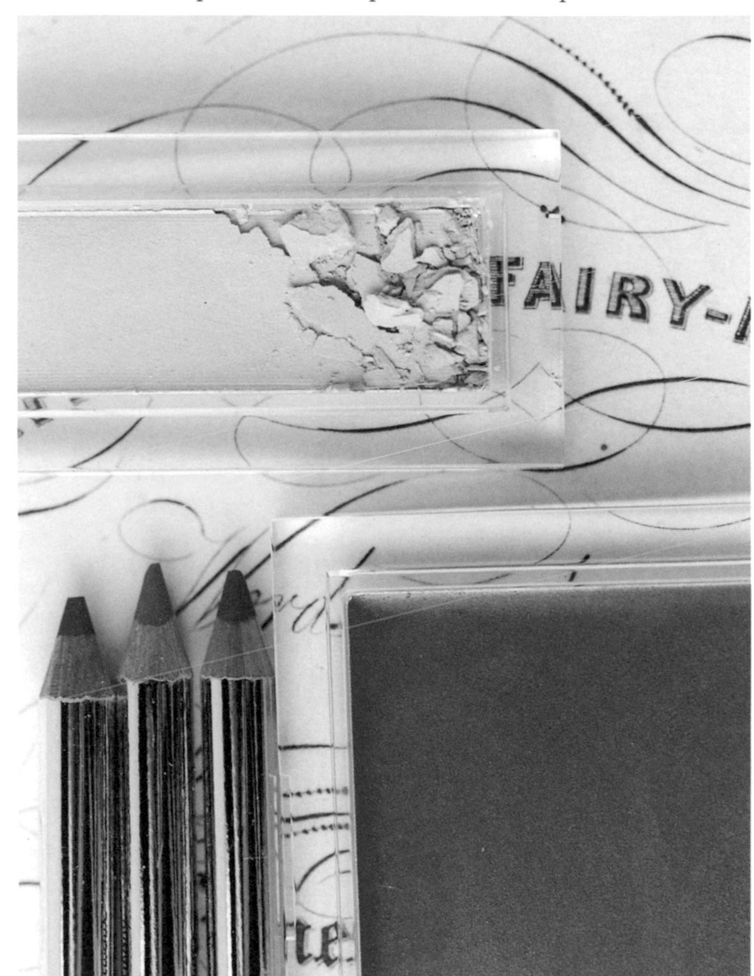

Blushes

Shadows

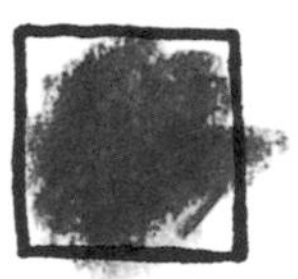

Lipsticks

brunette

BRUNETTE: If you're a brunette, chances are you have a tawny or yellow undertone in your skin and natural auburn highlights in your hair. Brunettes can look sallow without some extra color—a nice peachy blush, a reddish-brown lip color, and black mascara. The no-makeup look will wash you out. Go for corals and reds in the daytime with brown-black mascara; for nighttime glamour, intensify the color, groom your brows, change your mascara to black, and darken your lipstick.

If, on the other hand, you are a carbon copy of Snow White—dark brown hair that appears to be black; pale, ivory skin with pink undertones—play up the contrast. Wear very pale pink blush (if any at all) and deep blue-red lipstick. Don't line your eyes; instead, use several coats of very black mascara; groom and brush your dark brows, making sure they're not too thick or too close to your nose (which will make you look angry or sad).

Blushes

Shadows

Lipsticks

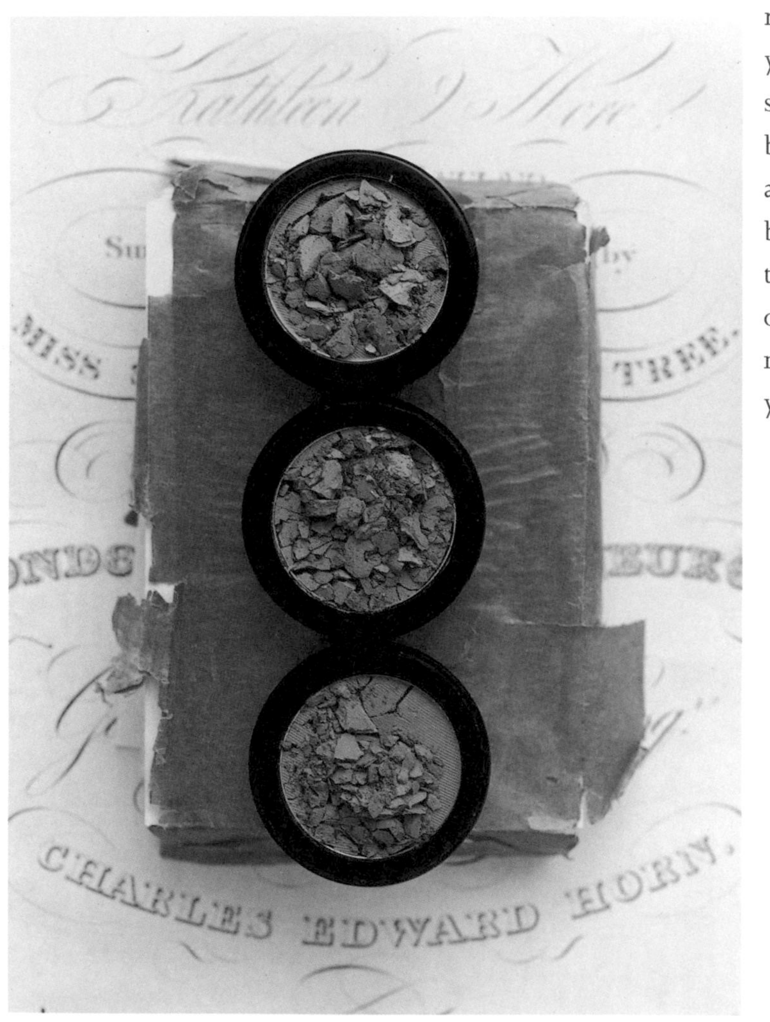

REDHEAD: If you're a natural redhead with pale skin and loads of freckles, always use a moisturizer with at least SPF 20, all day, every day—even on your hands. You can even out your skin tone with a light, sheer foundation that will allow your freckles to show through. Keep your skin warm and inviting with blushers that run from a delicate golden peach to a peachy brown. You can use bronze, brown, copper, sage, slate, burgundy, or gold on your eyes, with light brown mascara in the daytime and a darker shade with eyeliner at night. Your lip color can vary from shades of orange-red (yes, I know that I said orange never works, but if you have a lot of gold in your skin, on redheads it can look enchanting) and brown-red in the daytime, to deep burgundy or raisin shades for sexy drama at night.

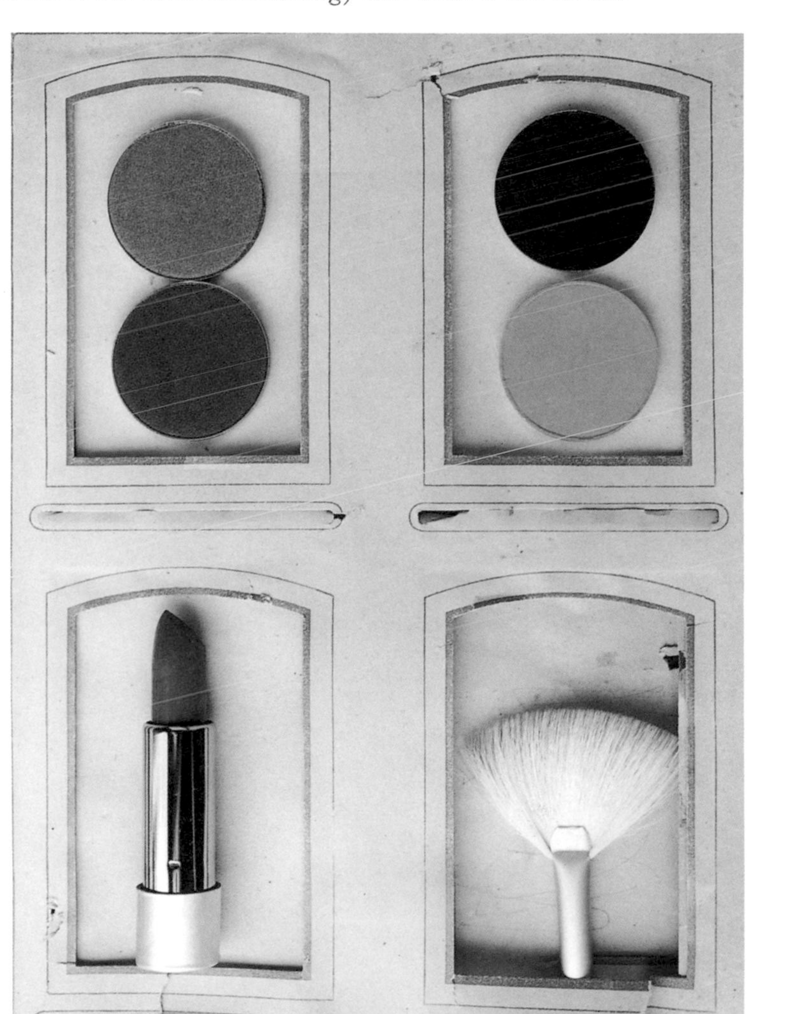

Blushes

Shadows

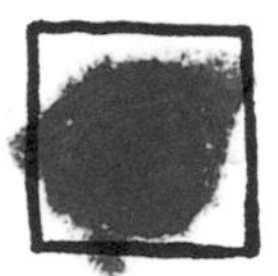

Lipsticks

african american

AFRICAN AMERICAN: Most likely you have either a red or a yellow undertone in your skin, which will determine the colors that look best on you. Regardless of your skin tone, stay away from cosmetics that have titanium dioxide in them. They tend to turn ashy on darker skins. Don't be afraid of using vivid, rich, deep colors like red or burgundy lipsticks and cream blushers that add highlights to your skin. Groom your eyebrows (African American women can have very sparse brows) with a dark pencil. On your lids, use matte shadows in shades of chestnut, brown, burgundy, or mahogany, or go all out and shimmer them up with copper, gold, bronze, and platinum. Always use a glossy black mascara.

Blushes

Shadows

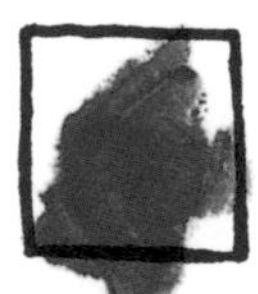

Lipsticks

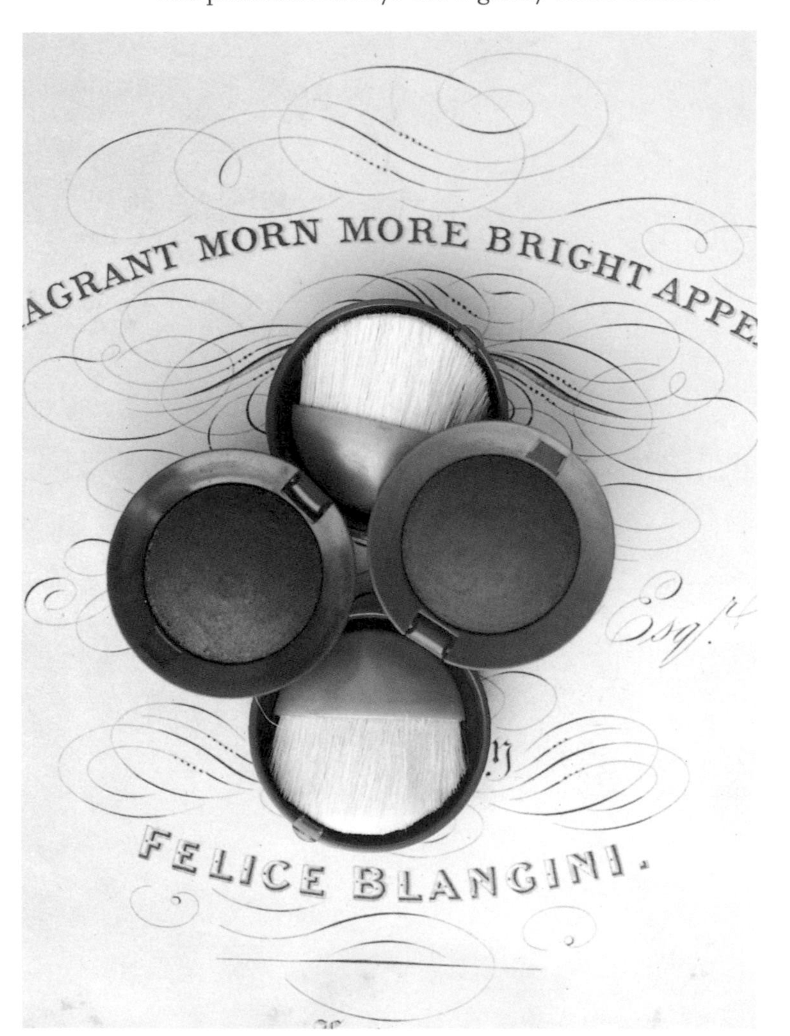

asian

ASIAN: To match your skin tone, find a foundation that disappears into your skin; most likely, it will have definite yellow tones in it. Your eyes need definition, as do your eyebrows if they are sparse and thin (you might consider having them dyed or augmented with permanent color; that is, tattooing). For a dramatic look, line your eyes with liquid liner all the way around and use an eyelash curler. Shiseido's curler has been designed for Asian eyes and will not pinch. Use a glossy black mascara that has a coating, not a building, formula, and practice applying it to the root of the lash for a thicker, more luxuriant look. Use plum, burgundy, or a rose/mauve blusher. Your lipsticks should have a little brown, rose, or mauve in them. Silvery mauves look very dramatic on you. For night: a deep red lipstick with theatrically dark eyes.

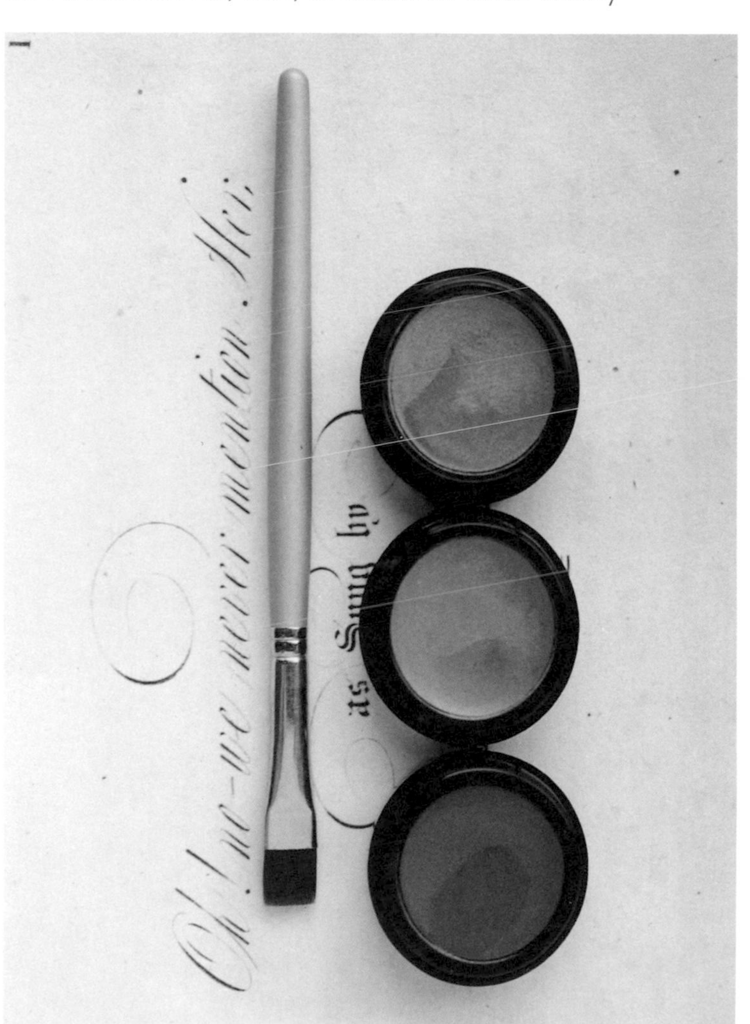

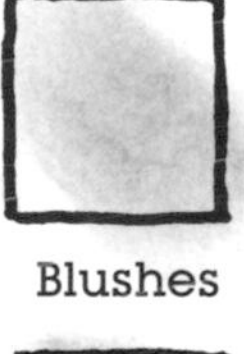

Blushes

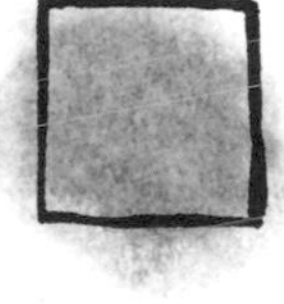

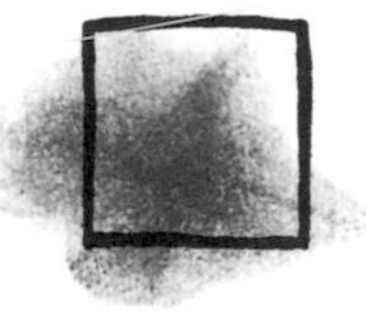

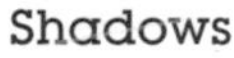

Shadows

Lipsticks

hispanic

HISPANIC: Don't mask your tawny skin tone with pinky foundation, because no amount of blending will ever make it look like anything but a mask. Find a good matching foundation with a yellow/tawny undertone but avoid dark makeups that turn orangey. Cosmetics in the strong coffee-cinnamon-brown range look great with your tawny skin and dark eyes. Use a blusher with burgundy or brown in it. You can wear chocolate browns and dark mahogany reds on your lips; for evening, try burgundy and plum shades. Pink will fade right into your skin, fuchsia will look harsh, and orange will look clownlike. If you've been blessed with thick, long, glossy lashes, your eyes probably don't need lining, but wear mascara—glossy black.

Blushes

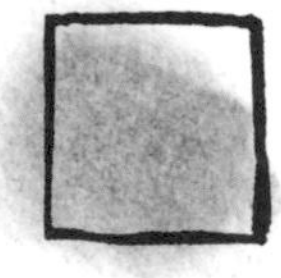

Shadows

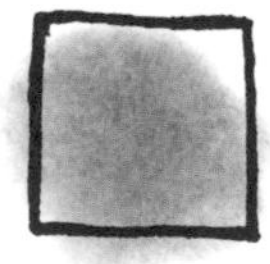

Lipsticks

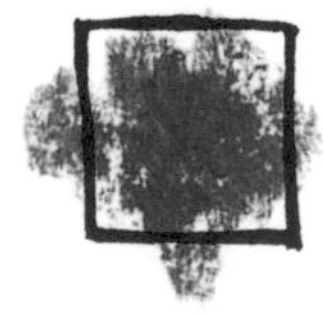

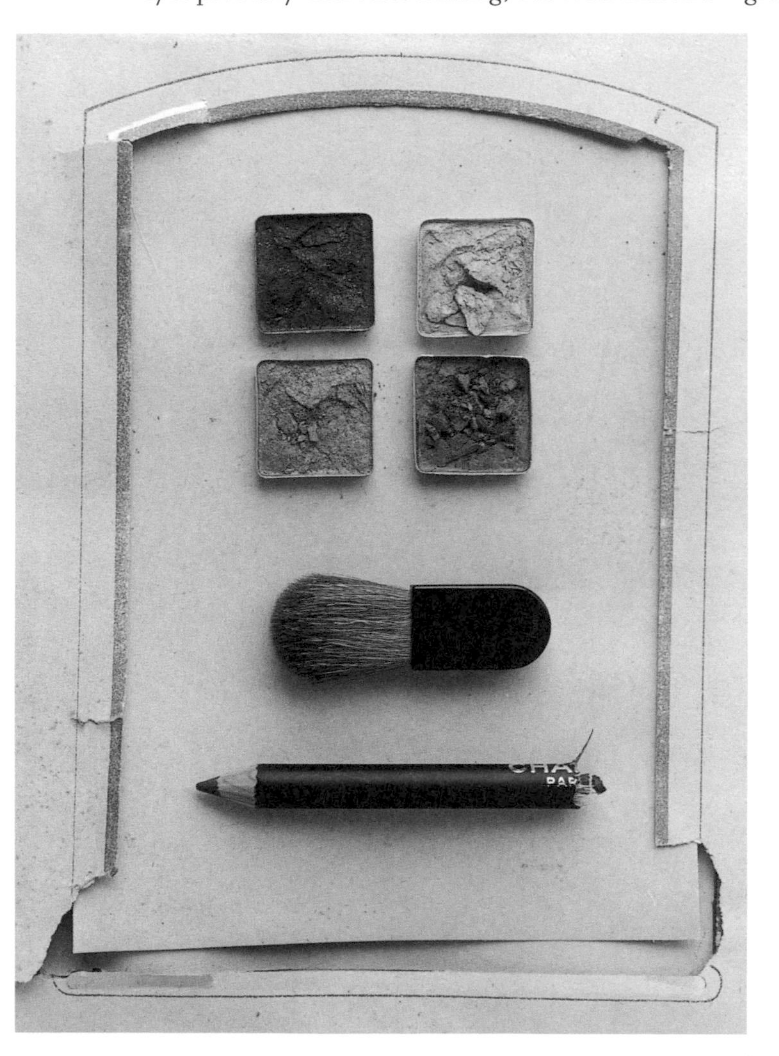

AGING: Less can always look like more. Lighten up your hand when you stroke on foundation. The aim here is to even skin tone, not mask it. You might want to try one of the new light-refracting premakeup moisturizers alone or under your foundation, or one of the latest light-refracting foundation formulas. Avoid colored finishing powders or powders with an excess of glimmer in them—they tend to settle in fine lines. Avoid pulling the skin around your eyes. If you want eyeliner, learn to use the brush/shadow method of dip and press, dip and press. Avoid lining under your eyes; it could emphasize dark circles. Find a waxy lip pencil that will prevent your lipstick from wandering. Matte lipsticks can both age and dry your lips. To brighten your face, choose a lively pink, peach, or red and apply it carefully with a brush to keep it from feathering.

SIMPLE MAKEUPS

Makeup does not require hours to apply. Most professionals tell you: If you can't do it quickly, don't bother. The idea is to enhance, not mask—so a light touch with the correct products can make even the most naturally maquillaged face look finished and pretty.

The Three-Minute Special: A Minimalist Approach

Say you've overslept. Or you have errands to run. You've just left the gym and are meeting a friend for coffee. In other words, you do not need a full makeup job, but you want to look presentable and finished. This makeup is geared to get you up and out in three minutes flat.

1. Apply moisturizer, sunscreen and concealer.
2. Even out skin with a light touch of foundation (here's where a cream-to-powder compact foundation comes in handy).
3. Apply mascara, two coats if you have the time.
4. Use a sheer lipstick, stain, or tinted gloss.

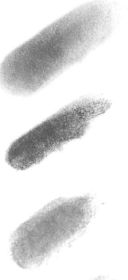

The Five-Minute Makeup: No Muss, No Fuss

If you are a professional woman and the day ahead of you is filled with conferences, meetings, and lunch out, you may want a more finished look, which will require a few more products and a less slapdash approach.

① Apply moisturizer, sunscreen, and foundation.

② Set foundation with a fluff of translucent powder.

③ Brush eyebrows, darken them with powder, and fix them with clear mascara or a gel-like brow fixative.

④ Line eyes; dust neutral shadow over lids from lash to crease.

⑤ Apply two coats of mascara. Use comb, brush, or spoolie to remove excess.

⑥ Line your lips and fill in with a brush if you can do it quickly; otherwise, use lipstick straight from the tube.

⑦ Apply blusher. Plop the center of the brush perpendicularly onto the blusher; shake off the extra, or dust it on the back of your hand; then fluff the brush over the apple of your cheek. Blend up and out with a velour puff.

⑧ Splash on scent, and you are ready to go.

The Evening Face: All about Intensity

Under artificial light or by candlelight at night, makeup can be more vivid and more dramatic. Colors can be darker; cheeks can appear more daringly angular; black mascara (or even fake lashes) is a must. You want your face to be mysterious, glamorous, striking. Night invites fantasy. It's time to play.

① Apply eye cream and moisturizer.

② Apply foundation, which can be heavier for evening. Choose one with more coverage, which will look like velvet under low-intensity lights or candlelight.

3. Use concealer over foundation in this instance to correct imperfections and to even out foundation, blending well with a sponge.
4. Use either pencil or the brush/shadow combination on your brows. Coat with clear mascara or brow-fix.
5. You can go darker on your lips for evening, either a more intense version of your favorite color or a shade of red complimentary to your skin tone. To get a precise line for a dramatic lip, line your lips first, then fill in the rest of the color with a lipstick brush.
6. Try a darker shade of cheek color for evening and concentrate on making your cheekbones stand out in bold relief by using the darker blush slightly under the apex and a shimmery highlighter on top to catch the light.
7. Set your makeup if you're out for a long evening by fluffing a sheer layer of translucent powder over the entire face. Use a clean powder brush to remove excess.

Enhancing Your Makeup Experience

- **Put your makeup on in very good light.** A well-lighted bathroom is good; diffused natural light is better. Avoid making up in full sunlight.
- **Update your makeup periodically to keep from looking as if you were perma-plaqued in time.** It can be something as simple as a new lipstick formula or a different way of wearing lipstick or blusher. Consider an addition to your makeup wardrobe as you would a new pair of shoes or a pretty scarf—something that will add some extra punch to your style.
- **Reserve one night or afternoon a week for your own personal home spa.** Indulge in a bubble bath with

some candles and privacy. Wash out your makeup brushes and sponges. Plant a couple of circles of fresh-cut cucumber rounds on your eyes and slather your favorite mask on your face. Spend that day out of makeup. Give yourself a well-deserved break.

- **Use a light touch**—literally—when applying makeup. Avoid stretching your eyelids as you stroke on eyeliner; don't scrub blusher into your cheeks. Use your ring finger to apply creams and cosmetics near the tender skin around your eyes.

Mistakes to Avoid

- **Hiding behind your foundation.** Masks keep people out, as they hide the real you. Use foundation to enhance, not to hide.
- **Gilding the lily.** Too much makeup is less attractive than not enough.
- **Wearing the same makeup that you did at 20.** Update your makeup and avoid looking as if you were fixed in amber at a time you thought you looked your best. Update. Update. Update.
- **Archiving your makeup.** Replace it often. Cosmetics don't last forever, especially foundations and mascara. If it smells, flakes, or separates, get rid of it.
- **Making your eyebrows too thin.** Few women have the sophistication and attitude necessary to look like Marlene Dietrich, circa 1933. Thin eyebrows look hard, tough, and dated. Plus, they require constant upkeep.
- **Matching eye shadow and lip color to clothes.** Good makeup compliments your skin tone, not your favorite fuchsia or turquoise dress. You can always find a lipstick that will highlight your features and not clash with your outfit.

HOW LONG SHOULD I KEEP MAKEUP?

Like eggs, spices, and milk, cosmetics will not last forever. And though there is no expiration date on them, they do lose their effectiveness at some point.

Cream blush. **Shelf life: two and one-half years**. Be sure to keep it tightly closed so the oils will not dry out or the product will crack.

Eyelash curler. **Shelf life: unlimited**. It's best to replace the rubber in it if it cracks or looks old. Clean your eyelash curler when you wash your brushes, about once a week.

Lipstick. **Shelf life: three to four years.** When a lipstick starts smelling waxy like a crayon, it's time to toss it.

Liquid Foundation. **Shelf life: six months to one year**. Toss it if it starts to smell funny or rancid, or if the color has separated. You can store your foundation in the refrigerator to extend its life, but you should warm it up considerably in your hands before you put it on your face.

Makeup Brushes. **Shelf life: unlimited.** If you keep them clean, they can last you a lifetime.

Mascara. **Shelf life: three months.** Mascara should be the most disposable of all your cosmetics, because it's prey to bacteria buildup. It will also start to dry out if you keep it too long.

Moisturizer. **Shelf life: one and one-half to three years**. Moisturizers will oxidize and bacteria will grow in it if you've dipped dirty fingers into it. To lengthen its life, use a cotton swab to dip the right amount out of the bottle onto your hand or face.

Nail Polish. **Shelf life: one and one-half to two years.** Nail polish always seems to thicken up when there is about half a bottle left. With a mini-bottle, you may be able to use up the polish before it thickens. Nail polish solvent or a small amount of polish remover can thin out thickened polish.

Pressed Cosmetics. **Shelf life: three years.** Eye Shadow, Blusher, Powder.If these products have any cream or oil in them, they will start to dry

Rule of Thumb:

Trust your sense of smell. If something smells like it's mildewed or rancid, it's time to throw it away.

out, lose their silkiness, and become difficult to blend after about three years. There is always a chance, also, of bacterial buildup on old pressed-powder cosmetics.

Sunscreen. Shelf life: one season. Some experts say two years, but after a season of lying on the deck or sand in direct sunlight, the chemical components in the sunscreen will start to break down. It's smart to start the sun season with fresh product.

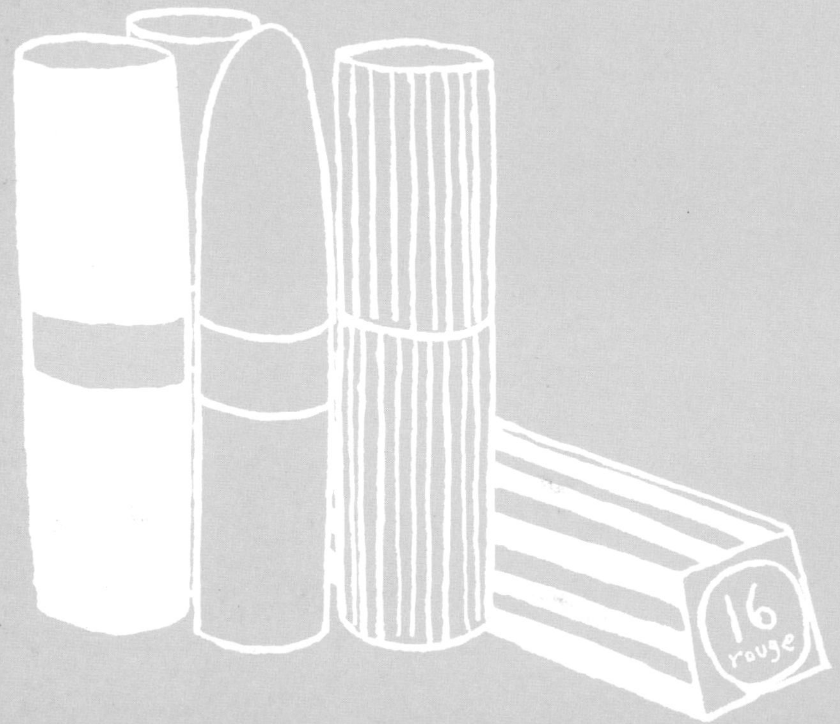

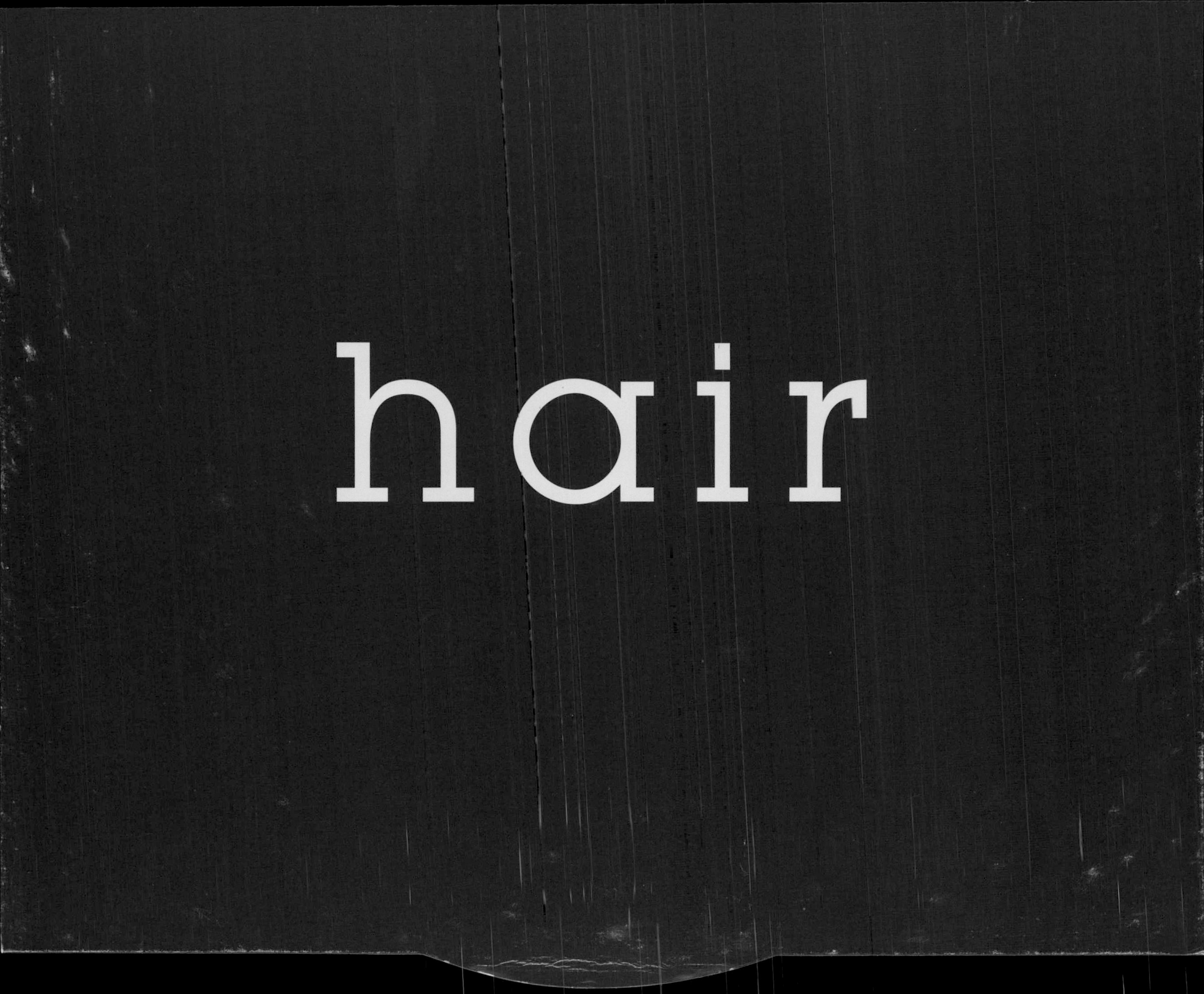
hair

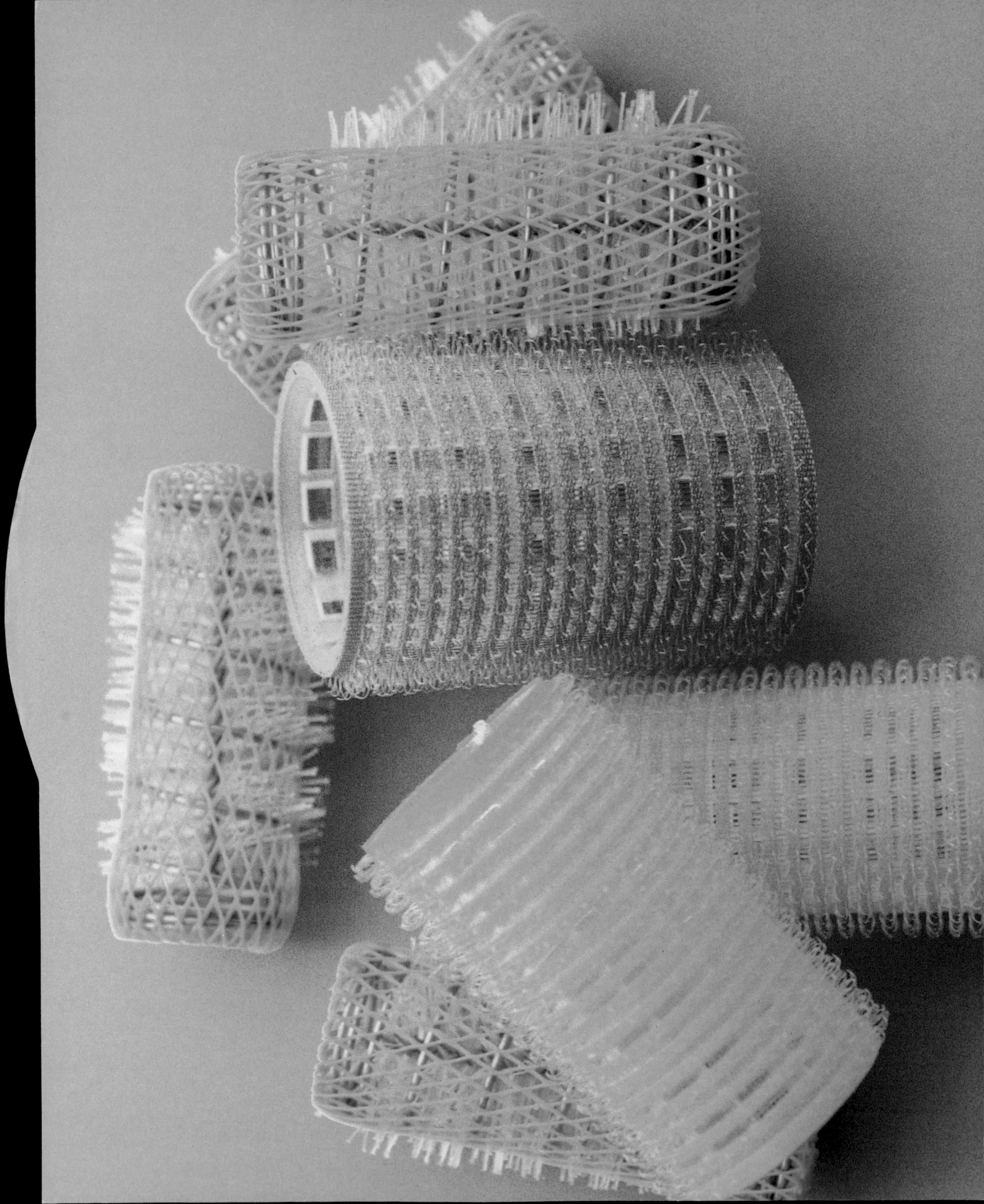

CHAPTER FOUR: HAIR

There is something about a woman's hair that prompts poets to take pen to paper and express the obvious. There is no ignoring what the Bible called a woman's "crowning glory." But sometimes, hair is not so glorious. Talk to ten women and, chances are, eight of them would rather have different hair. The curlies want straight, the straights want waves, and the thins want thick. Add to this dissatisfaction an occasional bad hair day, and it's not surprising that a growth industry has sprouted around women's displeasure with what their genes have brought them.

If I were going to purchase stock, I would probably invest in a company that sells hair products. Perhaps nothing in the cosmetic industry is growing quite as fast as hair—literally and figuratively. Toward the end of the twentieth century, women spent $42 billion on hair products annually. They not only wanted clean hair, but they also wanted it thicker, longer, softer, straighter, brighter, and more manageable. To that end, they bought volumizers, thickeners, growth stimulators, mousses, gels, tints, sprays, perms, and straighteners.

There is a common misconception that men get their hair genes from their mothers. That's just one of those old wives' tales about hair. A second misconception is that hair is a living organism that can be, in the carefully worded spiels of ad writers everywhere, "nourished." Hair is dead. Period. End of story. Once that hair shaft pops through the scalp, it is nothing but a collection of carefully arranged, but quite inanimate, keratin or protein cells. Hair develops from the same substance that forms claws and hoofs in animals, feathers on birds, scales on fish, and fingernails on humans. Organically, it is a combination of carbon, oxygen, hydrogen, nitrogen, and sulfur. There is nothing you can do, short of wearing a wig, that will change the structure, texture, and number of hairs on your head in any permanent manner. You can dye it, spray it, straighten it, and perm it, but when it grows out, it will be the same old hair you started with.

For better or worse, your parents have passed on their genes, which have given you your body type, eye color, skin tone, and hair quality (be it wavy, kinky, straight, or curly), its color, texture, and elasticity.

My Hair Won't Do What I Want

At a very early age, girls learn the limitations of their own hair—what it can, can't, will, and won't do. I was born with silky, wavy auburn hair, which, though there was a lot of it, was thin and flyaway. Debbie, my best friend in elementary school, had thick, blonde braids—heavy hair that hung golden and straight, like a curtain of wheat. There was no way that I was ever going to have hair that long, that thick, or that straight.

The only time I ever had the thick, luxuriant hair I longed for was in the mid-1960s when fake hair pieces—falls, wiglets, and switches—were in vogue. I can't think of any of my friends who, during that period, didn't resemble Alice in Wonderland with a long, glossy fall of hair attached at the crown of her head and tied with a pretty satin ribbon. Since then, I have realized that time is a more important commodity than long hair. So I've kept my hair clipped fairly short in a style I can whip up in 10 minutes. Any more than that, and I would be living in the beauty salon.

I grew up in the 1950s when hair was all about having someone else do it for you. Styles of the period—the bouffant, the beehive, and even the fluffy, face-framing artichoke made popular by Gina Lolobrigida—required salon visits, roller sets, at least half an hour under the dryer, followed by hair-damaging teasing to get the hair to do what it was never meant to do. Up-dos, chosen by every high-school girl who ever wanted elaborate prom hair, required about half a can of hair spray and tons of hairpins that carved canals in the scalp. Then along came Vidal Sassoon, and the entire zeitgeist of hair changed.

When Britisher Sassoon invented the precision cut in the late 1950s, he worked on hair types that would show off his painstaking shapes. Sassoon took women out of stiffly lacquered bouffants and beehives and into styles where hair was designed to fall back into place with a shake of the head. His best models—Peggy Moffitt and actress Nancy Kwan—had thick, glossy, straight, coarse hair. Try to put his classic five-point cut on someone with a slight wave and you get a funny-looking hybrid that was anything but chic or, for that matter, easy to care for.

Eventually, Sassoon did modify his cutting techniques to include hair that waved or curled naturally. When he clipped Mia Farrow's blonde tresses into a gamine cut that was no more than 2 inches at its longest point, women everywhere cut their hair.

Sassoon showed women that instead of becoming slaves to their hairdressers, they would owe a debt of gratitude to their haircutters. It was an obvious distinction that allowed women to have wash-and-wear hair, and visit the beauty shop every six to eight weeks for a trim.

Still women persist, panting after styles their hair will not support. In their quest for the hair they haven't, women have damaged what they have with blow-dryers, hot rollers, curling irons, products heavy in alcohol, abusive brushes, overcoloring, overstraightening, and overperming. There is only so much one little hair shaft can stand before it splits and frizzes. The cure: Cut the darn stuff off. And begin again.

ALIVE, ALIVE . . . OH!

In the beginning, hair *is* alive. The hair shaft grows from the follicle, a pocketlike structure, deep in the dermis. There are 5 million hair follicles on the human body; between 90,000 and 140,000 of them are on your head. At birth, the number of hairs on your head has been determined. If you're a Scandinavian blonde, you have the most hairs—up to 140,000. Brunettes are born with 110,000; and redheads, whose hair shafts are the thickest in diameter, have only 90,000.

There are four types of hair texture:

- **Straight.** Straight hair has absolutely no curl or wave. It can be baby fine and limp, or thick and coarse, which is common for Asians and Native Americans.
- **Wavy.** Hairdressers love to work with wavy hair. Although it stays close to the scalp when it grows out, it is easier to curl than straight hair, and its raggedness gives it more body, pliability, and thickness.

- **Curly.** Women with unruly mops of hair seem to be obsessed with controlling it. This is very high-maintenance hair that will curl or even frizz with the slightest rain or high humidity. Volume is difficult to predict or manage.
- **Kinky.** Frizzy and spiraled, kinky hair is prone to breakage because it has the fewest layers of protection and every bend of the curl has an inherent weakness. Kinky hair benefits from conditioning. It needs very little combing except a lift once in a while with a pick. It grows so dense that it can trap natural oils and dead skin cells close to the scalp, so it must be rinsed or washed regularly.

Your hair will change in texture and color from the time you are born until your early teens. Once you've gone through puberty, the hair you have is the hair you will keep for the rest of your life. You may get gray and, in the case of men, experience male-pattern baldness, but your growth patterns will remain the same.

Like every cell in your body, hair has a specific growth cycle. At any given time, hairs on your body are growing, resting, dormant, or sloughing off. The hairs on your head are no different. Were you never to cut your hair, in four to six years, it could grow to the length of three feet.

SHAFT: THE ANATOMY OF A HAIR

Hair, dead or not, is pure protein called keratin, which is formed by amino acids linking together in a chain called a peptide bond. Keratin has a high sulfur content and any chemical process—whether perms, straighteners, or peroxide-based colors—works by manipulating the sulfur bonds in the hair shaft.

Were you to examine a hair under a high-powered microscope, you would see not a solid length, but a series of colorless, transparent, over lapping shingle- or scalelike structures of keratin, which form the *cuticle*. The

Sassoon showed women that instead of becoming slaves to their hairdressers, they would owe a debt of gratitude to their haircutters. It was an obvious distinction that allowed women to have wash-and-wear hair, and visit the beauty shop every six to eight weeks for a trim.

scales of the cuticle are colorless. The major part of the hair shaft, the *cortex* and the *medulla*, hold the natural color of hair. If the cuticle stays flat and undamaged, hair is considered healthy. Damaged cuticles give hair such problems as frizzies and split ends. Hair products are designed to manipulate the cuticle and, as such, are only temporary measures.

If you mistreat your hair by teasing, overbrushing, excessive heat (blow-dryers, hot rollers, or curling irons), or by using products with a high percentage of alcohol (which is very drying), the individual scales of the cuticle will stand up and separate. The effect: dullness, frizzies, and split ends. You can spray on products to make your hair gleam, and you can use a product to control the frizzies. But for split ends, there is but one cure: Cut them off.

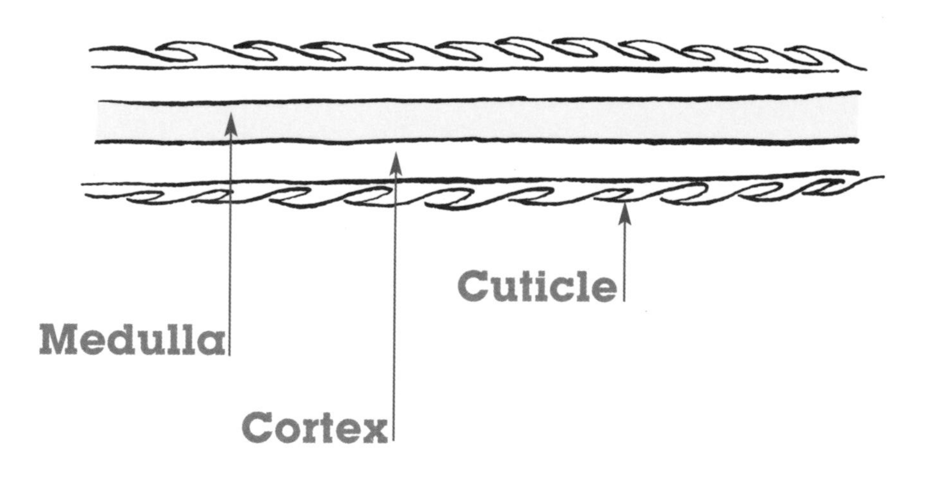

How Does My Hair Behave?

Your hair may be curly or straight, thick or thin, but to determine what type, rather than what texture, of hair you have, ask yourself the following:

1. **Does my hair require a minimum of attention?**
2. **Does my hair have good body? Is it soft to the touch?**
3. **Does my hair get oily the same day I wash it?**
4. **Does my hair cling to my scalp? Does it refuse to hold a style?**
5. **Is my hair harder to manage right before my period?**
6. **Do I have pimples on my forehead under my bangs?**
7. **Does my scalp itch?**
8. **Do I have little flakes of white on my collar and shoulders?**
9. **Does my hair have a lot of static and flyaway ends?**

Interpretation.

If you've answered yes to questions 1 and 2, you have normal hair. If you've answered yes to questions 3 through 6, you have oily hair. If you've answered yes to questions 7 through 9, you have dry hair.

Normal Hair. Perhaps "normal" is a misnomer. Maybe the word should be *natural,* hair in its ideal state. If your hair feels soft to the touch, has good body, is manageable, and has not been permed, straightened, or colored, it is in its natural state. Neither over-oily or too dry, this kind of hair needs minimal attention—probably a shampoo every two to three days. If you blow-dry your hair each morning, use a conditioner on the days you don't shampoo. If you color your hair or treat it with any kind of chemical solution, if you overstyle with products that contain alcohol, or if you use a blow-dryer or hot rollers too often, you can damage your hair.

Oily Hair. It is not your hair that is oily (hair is dead, remember?) but your scalp that is producing too much sebum, or, natural oil, which can make your hair feel lank, flat, and greasy. If you have oily hair, you probably wash your hair every day; but be careful. Strong shampoos designated for oily hair can have too much detergent, which can dry out the scalp and hair; this will signal the oil glands to start pumping out more oil.

Changes in hormone levels (when you're expecting your period, pregnant, menopausal) can also affect the amount of sebum your scalp produces. If you are pregnant, your hair may be extremely oily because your body is producing enough hormones to allow you to carry to term. And when your period ceases, your hormone levels drop, and you may wake up some morning with hair that has a whole new set of problems or assets.

Dry Hair. Dry hair tends to be fine and thin. Your scalp feels itchy and produces a lot of dead skin cells that look like dandruff on your dark clothes after you've brushed your hair. Dandruff-like conditions come from dead-skin-cell buildup, where cells have not had the opportunity to slough off. This can be caused by overusing conditioners, not washing your hair often enough, not rinsing thoroughly, using products with a high alcohol content, or accumulating styling gels or sprays on the hair shaft. (Dandruff is another condition altogether. It is thought to be the product of a yeast organism, which exists naturally on the scalp but has gotten out of control.)

Beauty Tip 17: Treat dry scalp as you would dry skin. Use a lightweight moisturizer like Cetaphil on the scalp overnight for treatment; wash it out well in the morning.

HELP! I'M HAVING A BAD HAIR DAY

Regardless of the quality of your cut, the excellence of your products, and the skill you have with your hair, once in a while, your hair is simply going to look awful. Bad hair days are just part of life. However, they don't just come out of the blue. They happen when:

- **Your styling products have built up in your hair.**
- **Your hair is really clean** (clean hair is much harder to manage than day-old hair that has a little dirt in it).
- **Your hormones vary**—the week before your period, increased estrogen can accelerate oil production and create greasy hair.
- **Changes occur in your normal environment.**

Have you ever noticed, for instance, how great your hair looks when you step onto a plane, and how awful it looks and feels when you get off? The lack of humidity in airplane air causes the moisture in your hair to evaporate, and even the best style will collapse. And, if you have moved from California to, say, Ohio, you might see a change in the behavior of your hair. Where it once almost jumped through hoops for you, it refuses to stay down and behave in another city. Humidity, dryness, quality of the water, and change in season can affect the porosity (ability to hold moisture) of your hair. Dryness can make your hair flyaway and unmanageable; humidity will cause your hair to curl or frizz.

There is not much you can do about a bad hair day short of wetting your hair and starting over, or calling the hair salon to see if they can work you in. Many unnecessary haircuts have come from impatience generated by bad hair days. Calm down, try to restyle, and when in doubt, plop on a chic little hat and forget about it.

Beauty Tip 18: Another minor cause of bad hair days: That phone call in the middle of your styling routine. If you allow your hair to dry before you've finished styling it, redampen your hair and start all over.

THE TAMING OF THE MANE: THE RIGHT TOOLS AND PRODUCTS

Men have it easy. They can usually get away with wet-combing their hair into place and letting it dry. Women's lives, and hair, are much more complicated. A comb and brush is simply not enough. At any given time, you could probably find enough hair product and gizmos in a cabinet under the sink, in the linen closet, or on the dresser to open your own store. But here are the basic tools that many hairdressers recommend for home use.

Beauty Tip 19:
To increase the volume of your hair, blow-dry it against the direction it grows; hot air creates more volume by opening the cuticle layers. There is one problem: This method also increases the number of fly-away hairs.

Power Tools

Blow-dryers. The dryer is your primary styling tool. A good one will balance comfortably in your hand and not be too heavy. It should have at least 1,200 watts, but the pros like dryers with 2,000 watts. There should be an assortment of settings, including a cool-down button to keep the dryer from getting too hot. The straight-nozzle dryer will direct the heat where you want it; just don't use it too close to your hair—3 to 6 inches away is the recommended distance. Make sure the dryer has a fairly long cord so you can change hands and direction without pulling the plug.

Most dryers come with attachments. The round, perforated disk, a diffuser, distributes the air in a cooler, wider manner and is excellent for naturally curly hair or for scrunching hair to make it look curly. A lifting comb allows the air to get under the hair at scalp level.

To use a dryer properly, wrap your hair around a brush and allow the air from the dryer to go up and over, and underneath, the brush.

Hot Rollers. Use on dry (that is, not wet) hair only. Plug-in rollers are the fastest way to give your hair temporary curl or to revive a set. However, if they are used too often, their dry heat can damage hair.

Steam Rollers. These are gentler on the hair because they're usually made of soft foam, heated up in a canister containing boiling water. Steam-rolled sets are tighter and last longer.

Curling Iron. The age-old method of curling hair—by wrapping it around a heated metal cylinder—became easier when curling irons were electrified. Use a curling iron on dry (not wet) hair only. A good iron has more than one heat setting and does not get hot at the tip. The clamp that holds the hair should open and close easily and not snag the hair. You can find irons in different circumferences for loose or tight curls, long or short hair.

Non-Power Tools

A good brush used in conjunction with a blow-dryer and styling products can make the difference between a good style and a mediocre one. Make sure you choose the correct size brush for the hair style you have. For example, do not attempt to use a small-circumference brush on long hair. It just won't work.

All-Purpose Half-Round Brush. This is the most common styling brush that you can use with a blow-dryer or for simply brushing hair into place. Find a brush with soft, natural bristles or with pliable plastic bristles that are not set too close together.

Round Brush. This brush is available in many different circumferences and is used with blow-dryers to curl or lift the hair. The brush acts as an instant hair roller when you wrap your hair around it. Some round brushes have natural bristles; others have plastic bristles set into metal cores that heat up with blow-drying and function as a very large roller.

Vent Brush. A slightly curved half-brush, a vent has plastic bristles tipped with tiny balls. The bristles are set fairly wide apart and are excellent for working through wet hair that has been conditioned or sprayed with a detangler. Also, you can use this brush while drying your hair for some lift and fullness.

Flat-Paddle Brush. This has wire or nylon bristles set into a rubber cushion in a flat, oval, or square base. It is used with a blow-dryer for pulling the curl out of long or curly hair.

Beauty Tip 20: If you want a super-straight hairdo, try brushing your wet hair around your head as if it were a massive roller as you blow-dry, being careful not to hold the dryer too close. The resulting style will allow the hair to fall straight.

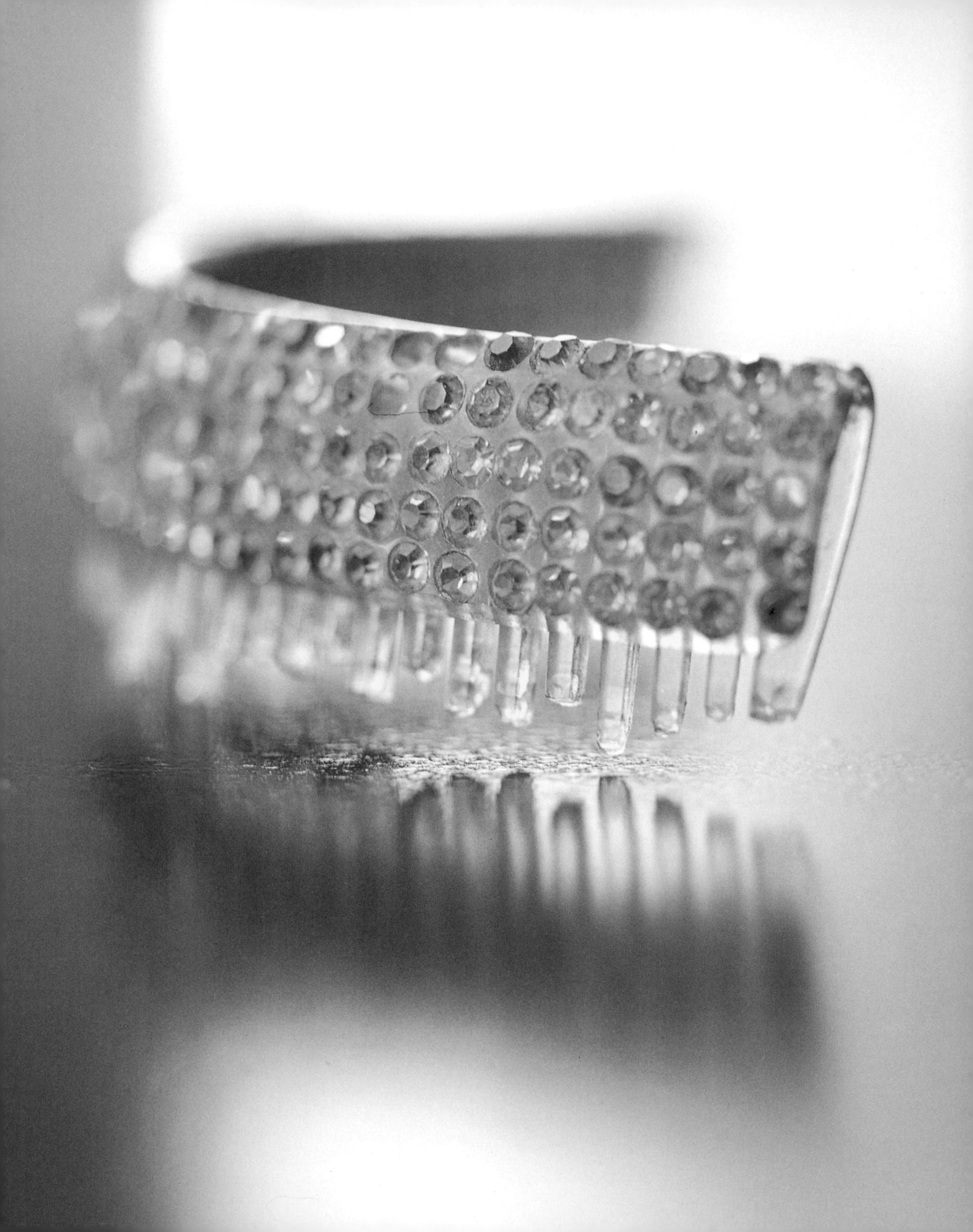

Combs

A man's comb is his styler, and it usually gets carried in a breast or back pocket. But a woman has many different types of combs in her arsenal, the least of which is for neatening up her hair during the day.

Fork Comb and Pick. Usually plastic, but sometimes metal, this double-ended tool has a comb with alternating, variably sized teeth on one end, and a four-pronged metal pick at the other for back-combing then lifting the hair.

Rattail Comb. With teeth set closely together and a long, tapered handle, this is a finishing or styling comb designed to smooth and lift the hair.

Wide-Toothed Comb. Usually 5 or 6 inches long and 2 inches deep with large, very wide-set teeth, this comb is used on wet, just-shampooed hair or for distributing gel through the hair.

Pick. A heavy plastic forklike tool with long tines set wide apart, a pick is used to lift curly or kinky hair that has become matted during sleep or flattened by a hat, scarf, or humidity.

Miscellaneous Styling Aids

For every kind of hair style, there are gizmos designed to help get you there, from numerous sized and shaped rollers to hair clips, headbands, elastic bands, and pins.

Self-Stick Rollers. Designed to hold the hair in place without bobby pins, these have tiny rough spikes on the surface to keep hair from slipping. If pulled out of the hair roughly, they can add to cuticle breakage.

Sponge Rollers. These are great for making spiral curls. You can use them with wet or damp hair under a salon hair dryer. They're soft enough to sleep on, so you can set your hair before bedtime and allow it to dry overnight.

Bendable Stick Rollers. Wind long hair around these and bend them to lock in place. They're great for the fashionable long-haired wavy or gently curled Rapunzel look. Simply take hair out of the curlers, fluff it slightly with your fingers, and let it hang down.

Beauty Tip 21:
To give your hair some lift, you may want to tease it or back-comb, an effective technique for building body into hair. Take a section of hair and run the comb gently up and down it, letting the hairs pile up on one another. To smooth hair over the top, use a light stroke of a half-brush. You can spray this arrangement and then gently lift from underneath with a rattail comb, or use the pick for even more lift. However, if you back-comb too vigorously or too often, you will damage the cuticle and cause breakage and frizzies.

Bobby Pins. Flat, springy pins, each one made from one piece of bent tempered metal with plastic tips, these hold hair in place. They're also good for fastening on a bow or flower. Available in short or long, these strong pins are used in elaborate swept-up styles, in French twists, or to fasten on hairpieces.

Hairpins. Thinner than bobby pins, hairpins—about 2 inches long—are each made from U-shaped wire. These are good when an invisible, light hold is needed.

Styling Clips. Spring-controlled, metallic hair clips were used in pin-curl hairstyles that required time under the dryer. In recent years, with the popularity of blow-dry/brush styling, they have gone out of vogue.

Wave Clips. These long, tapered clips each catch the ridge of a damp wave and hold it in place until it dries.

Alligator Clips. With a set of teeth arranged along each side of a spring-controlled fastener, these look a lot more dangerous than they are. Use them to clip long hair into a casual semi-ponytail if you want to avoid rubber bands or elastics.

Comb Coil. An alternative to the headband, this length of plastic teeth is designed to hold the hair back with some tension.

Elastics. These fabric-covered bands have bungee-cord-style ends that hook together to hold hair in a ponytail. Fabric-covered rubber bands, which reduce damage and hair breakage, are also called elastics.

CARING FOR YOUR CROWNING GLORY

Before you can even contemplate styling, cutting, coloring, or perming your hair, you should consider how best to take care of it—how to get it into the best shape possible. Were you to leave your hair alone—that is, just brush it enough to loosen dead skin cells at scalp level and wash it once a week to remove excess oil—your hair would do what nature intended it to do.

Drugstore shelves, however, are chockablock with products for people who are dissatisfied with what their hair would do if left to its own devices. You can buy all the straightening gels, volumizers, frizzies-smoothers, and hair sprays you want, but cosmetic expert Paula Begoun says, "There are no hair-care products that can repair, fix, correct, restructure, form, change, restore, rebuild, or alter damaged hair. Hair is dead; it cannot be repaired or added on to in any way."

Yet, it is possible to *temporarily* alter the behavior of your hair with modern products from cosmetic companies that have expensive research and development facilities behind them. That does not automatically mean that expensive salon products are necessarily any better than those you buy in the drugstore. Often the same cosmetic giants will field two different lines, one for salon and one for mass market, both of which benefit from the company's research and development.

HAIR-RAISING CLAIMS

There are certain bits of information about hair and hair products that are often repeated as fact, when they are not:

• **Expensive hair products are better than cheaper ones.** False.

You may get more personal service at your beauty salon, where there are fewer product lines to choose from, than from a drugstore whose acres of product-lined shelves can confuse and intimidate. But here's something you may not know: Your hairdresser may be on commission and promoting a certain product line. Also, 30 to 40 percent of his or her income is derived from selling product to clients (you).

• **Over-the-counter hair products encourage hair growth.** False.

According to the Food and Drug Administration, over-the-counter products are not supposed to have pharmaceutical capability. Only physician-prescribed and -supervised drugs like Minoxidil have been known to stimulate hair growth.

- **Every type of hair needs conditioning.** False.

Not everyone needs to use a conditioner. If your hair is dry or if you can't get a comb through it when it's wet, then use a detangler. Also, if you use a lot of heat on your hair—dryer, curling iron, or hot rollers—apply a conditioner to help protect the cuticle.

- **Hair has to squeak to be really clean.** False.

Hair will be squeaky clean if your water is hard and contains a lot of calcium deposits. Because most cities have hard water, squeaky-clean hair is pervasive.

- **I must brush my hair 100 strokes every night.** False.

That bit of old wives' tale comes down from our Victorian ancestors who did a lot of strange things (like undressing in the dark). You can do untold damage to the cuticle of your hair if you whip a brush through it 100 times a night. Brushing roughs up the hair and chips away at the cuticle, exposing the cortex to breakage and damage.

- **Drugstore hair color is not as good as salon color.** False.

Let me let you in on a little secret: Many hairstylists will actually use drugstore color if they like it better than what their salon stocks. If you are just trying to brighten your own hair color or refresh the one your salon has done, you can save a lot of money by using drugstore color. However, if you want a radical color change—like going from brunette to baby blonde—see your colorist.

WASHING, CONDITIONING, AND STYLING PRODUCTS

You could probably wash your hair with hand soap, but I wouldn't. Aesthetically, we've gotten used to nice-smelling, specially formulated products to care for our hair. What you choose is a matter of taste. Here's a sampling of what's out there.

Shampoos

Whether you buy a fancy expensive designer shampoo or a cheap generic bottle from the drugstore, chances are the ingredients are almost exactly the same. The shampoo is mostly water infused with a surfactant (short for *SURFace ACTive AgeNT*) says expert Paula Begoun, which actually does the heavy cleaning, and lather agents, humectant moisture-attractors, thickeners, preservatives, and this season's "miracle product." That could be vitamin E, collagen, citrus, menthol, oregano, basil, essential oil, mango extract, hemp, tea-tree oil, or awapuhi (extract of Hawaiian ginger). Chances are that those last ingredients are there in such small amounts that they are only window dressing or an advertising gimmick.

Shampoos can also contain volumizers (body builders) and hair thickeners such as glycerin, propylene glycol, panthenols, and proteins that cause the cuticle of the hair to swell. This means the hair shaft will look and feel thicker; and it will have gained instant volume.

If someone tells you that you should change your shampoo once in a while, it's probably good advice, not because your hair has become immune to the charms and attributes of your current shampoo, but rather, because it has built up in your hair, and only a slightly more detergent shampoo could strip the hair of everything. Remember, the purpose of a shampoo is to wash the hair and scalp to help clear away dead skin cells and natural oils, as well as buildup from the hair products you use.

Conditioners

Conditioners make the hair softer, shinier, silkier, and more combable right when its wet. Both rinse-off and leave-in conditioners are designed to coat the hair shaft and make the cuticle stay down. Conditioners may contain proteins like collagen or elastin, which coat the hair shaft but will not restructure it; amino acids that will rinse away; polysaccharides like glycerin, sorbitol, and butylene glycol; water binders for thickening and silkiness; and fatty acids called lipids, which add slip to the hair. Hair with a smooth cuticle shines, but if the conditioner is too heavy, hair can look lank, flat, and greasy.

Beauty Tip 22: When using any hair product for the first time, start off with a small amount. Experiment on a night when you don't have to go anywhere.

The jury is still out on vitamin B-complex derivatives (Panthenol and biotin, or any vitamin enrichment, for that matter) in shampoos and conditioners. They do have a proven affinity for the hair and actually penetrate the hair shaft. Panthenol does have some humectant properties that can give brittle hair needed swing and movement and add some shine.

The best new wrinkle in hair products is silicone—dimethicone cyclomethicone—which, when it clings to the surface of the hair cuticle, can affect the texture by adding smoothness and manageability. If your hair tends to be coarse, dry, or frizzy, start using products that have this ingredient.

You've probably bought shampoos and conditioners that claim to contain alpha-hydroxy acids (AHAs) and beta-hydroxy acids (BHAs). Again, these occur in such small quantities that they can't do anything. They are added to some shampoos to exfoliate the scalp, but you can accomplish that by simply scratching your head gently with your fingernails or by using a rubber scalp stimulator.

Hair Masks, Packs, Hot-Oil Treatments. Sometimes hair has been so damaged by overbrushing, overheating, or overprocessing (perming, straightening, tinting) that it needs intensive conditioning. These products have the same ingredients as regular conditioners, but in order to function, they require either time or heat.

Laminates, Serums, Hair Polishers. Designed to smooth away the frizzies and add shine, these products contain some form of silicone.

Pomades. Barber shops have been selling these petroleum products for years. They're really a form of mustache wax made from petrolatum, wax, mineral oil, lanolin, or castor oil and should be used only for special effects like making short hair stand on end or long hair bunch up in tight tendrils. They feel greasy and build up in the hair, attracting dust and dirt.

Styling Preparations

The nice thing about hair science of the past 50 years is that hair care companies have come up with products to help you achieve the look you want with a minimum of fuss.

Mousse. When you shake up the can, mousse comes out under pressure and looks like whipped cream in your hand. It contains a lot of air and alcohol and, ultimately, can be very drying to the hair. Used sparingly, it will improve a style by imparting fullness and body to the hair.

Gel. More viscous than mousse, gel gives more control and fullness when massaged into the roots of wet hair, which can then be blown dry. Gel can also be used to slick down hair for a dramatic, patent-leather look.

Hair Spray. Spray has the same ingredients as mousse and gel, just in a more concentrated form. Hair spray has more direct holding power. The alcohol and plasticizing agents that allow the fine mist to dry quickly can also damage dry, fine, or brittle hair. Sprays with a high alcohol content will also add insult to injury if hair is treated—colored or permed—or if the cuticle shows extreme damage (frizzies and split ends).

QUICK KITCHEN AID FOR HAIR

You do not have to spend a fortune on hair products if your kitchen is well stocked. Raid your pantry for a few of these organic treatments:

- **Strong Coffee.** If you are a brunette, you can enhance your color by rinsing your dry hair with strong coffee. Leave cooled coffee in for 30 minutes, then rinse out, dry, and style. Note the beautiful new highlights.
- **Cooled Chamomile Tea.** Spray dry hair with chamomile tea and leave it in for 20 minutes to liven up mousy brown or dishwater-blonde hair.
- **Flat Beer.** Pour flat beer into a clean spray bottle and mist damp hair before setting. The alcohol smell will not linger. Use beer to jazz up an exhausted perm or bring spring back to naturally curly hair.
- **Banana.** Mash fruit and add a few drops of almond oil. Massage it into your hair and scalp for instant first-aid for damaged or dry hair. Leave it on for 15 minutes and rinse out completely.

Beauty Tip 23: Buy trial-size bottles (like you get in hotel bathrooms) of products at beauty supply stores, and experiment until you find the right ones for you.

- **Aloe Vera.** Mix ½ cup of shampoo with ¼ cup of aloe-vera gel for a quick oily-hair treatment. Apply to hair, comb it through, and rinse out carefully.
- **Eggs and Honey.** For a dry-hair treatment, combine one egg with a teaspoon of honey and a tablespoon of olive oil; rub this mixture into wet hair and cover with a plastic shower cap. Leave it on for half an hour, then shampoo well.

MANIPULATING YOUR MANE

Dying for the Facts

Ask a woman why she colors her hair and you might get the following reasons:

- ***Because I'm getting gray.*** The largest segment of people who buy hair color these days want to cover gray. This includes both men and women.
- ***Because my hair tends to be thin and the dye adds body.***
- ***Because I'm bored.***
- ***Because I want the same color of hair that I had as a child.*** Ask a redhead, and chances are, she bemoans the fact that those coppery curls she had as a youngster have darkened and dulled with age.

Once you've made the decision to color your hair—for whatever reason—you have to determine what kind of color you want: something temporary to test out, or something more permanent that will take more than a week of shampooing to remove.

Temporary Color

If you're really curious but don't want to invest a lot of time or money, then temporary color is for you. Basically, it is a stain that involves only the surface of the hair.

Because of the nature of temporary colors (they lack peroxide and ammonia), you can manipulate only the *natural* color of your hair by a few intensities. Temporary color is also available in a hair mascara format, which is the easiest to experiment with because it washes out after one use. Very light mascaras are good for highlighting, and crazy hues like fuchsia, electric blue, neon green, and purple are available for special occasions. Temporary colors also come in shampoo, conditioner, and mousse formulations. They are very short lived and will wash out after one or two shampoos. The color is deposited onto the hair shaft, not into it. What you see in the container is what you'll get on your hair.

You can use temporary color to tone down the brassiness of blonde, to neutralize the yellow in white or gray hair, or to make your own color a bit more glossy and deep.

Semipermanent Hair Color without Peroxide

This type of color, also considered a stain because it works on the cuticle, not in the center of the hair shaft, is available in a cream, gel, mousse, or shampoo. It must be left on the hair for at least 20 minutes, and it will last through six or seven shampoos. Semipermanent color embeds itself in the cuticle but does not require ammonia to lift the cuticle or peroxide to bleach out your natural color. Semipermanent color can darken or brighten your natural color and blend away gray hairs. This is color with training wheels. Use it to see whether you really want to change the color of your hair—it's an experiment that requires little commitment because the dye washes out so quickly and leaves no regrowth to worry about.

Semipermanent Color with Peroxide

This kind of color is the longer lasting and requires a low concentration of peroxide and ammonia. You can use it to change from brunette to red, or from blonde to red, but it will not be effective for a drastic change, like brunette to blone. Also called demipermanent color, it covers gray more effectively than a stain. It requires heat and time (as much as 45 minutes) to develop.

Permanent Hair Color

There are two kinds of permanent hair color: single process and double process.

Single Process. This is a shampoo-in root application that has a minimal amount of ammonia and a low volume of peroxide. It is left on the hair for 20 to 45 minutes. In the initial application, the color is combed all the way through the hair to the ends. Single-process color produces roots that need to be touched up every four to five weeks with your color formula; touch-ups require the same amount of time as the initial coloring. The inherent problem with peroxide-assisted color changes is the danger of oxidation. Golds and reds will fade over time or will react chemically with the oxygen in the air. Reds will fade or oxidize to the undertones of the hair, namely orange, and golds will turn brassy and yellow. To keep this kind of color longer, tinted shampoos and conditioners will help, as will staying out of direct sunlight.

Double Process. If you were born a brunette and have always longed to be a blonde, be prepared for the rigors of two-step color. Like skin color, hair color depends upon the amount of melanin it contains. When you change your hair this radically, you have to first get to the cortex—that's where ammonia comes in. Ammonia causes the cuticle to splay and lift, baring the rest of the hair shaft, which facilitates the second process, reaching the melanin with bleach. The result is hair that resembles light-yellow straw: that is, hair without melanin. To achieve your new color—whether you want to be a baby blonde, a golden blonde, or bombshell platinum—a toner is applied that will recolor the melanin with your desired hue. After that, your colorist may want to put a clear glaze on your new color to protect it and to keep it shiny.

Blonde hair requires a lot of maintenance—from using tinted shampoos (blue for cooler blondes; golden for warmer blondes) to getting touch-ups on regrowth every three to four weeks. You might feel like you've started to keep company with your hairdresser or are, at least, putting his or her children or significant other through college.

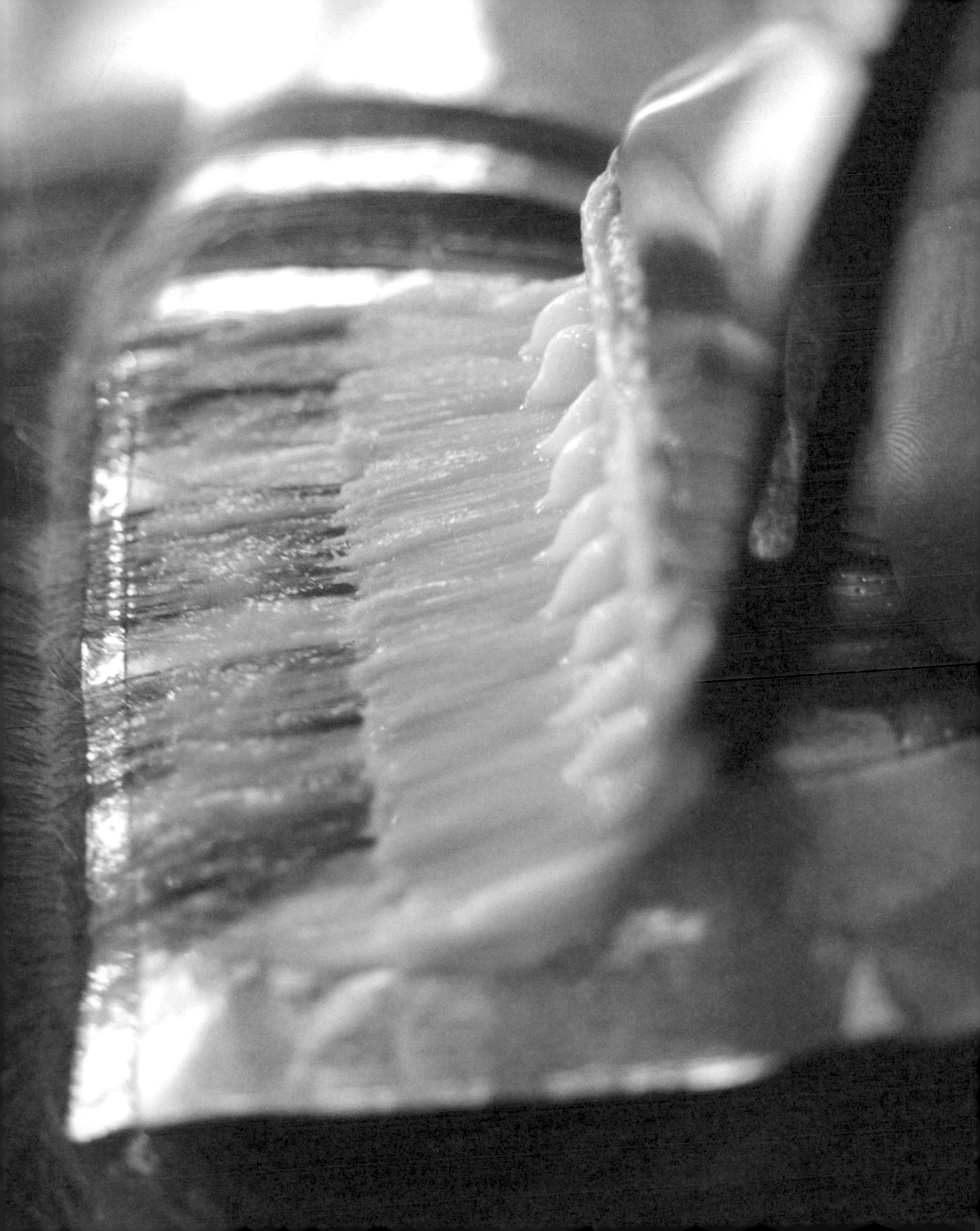

Highlighting

The best way to hide gray or be "sort of" blonde or "sort of" red is to have highlights added to your natural hair color. By *highlighting,* I mean separating out certain sections of your hair with a comb and applying bleach and permanent color to them. Highlights can be applied using several different techniques for a variety of effects.

Weaving. You've seen women in beauty salons wearing foil packets all over their heads, as if they were trying to phone Venus. This process is very labor-intensive and takes a long time. A full head of woven highlights can cost as much as $300 if your hair is long or if you live in New York or Los Angeles, where things are more expensive.

When highlights are woven in, the colorist takes a thin segment of hair and weaves a rattail comb in and out until a tiny amount of hair is separated. These will be painted with a bleaching solution and then wrapped in foil to separate them from the rest of the hair. Sometimes, colorists will apply different hues of blonde, darker and lighter, to each row of hair to give hair more depth and variation or a more natural, sun-lightened appearance. When processing is finished, the bleach is washed out of the hair, and a toner is added. Woven highlights require touch-ups only about three times a year because they don't show much regrowth.

Painting or Baliage. As with weaving, the aim here is to make hair look as if it had been sun-streaked naturally. This free-hand method is less precise, and the outcome is not predictable. In this process, color is applied to random sections of the hair with a comb or a brush dipped in the color solution. Sometimes the color-treated hair is covered with plastic wrap, squished down to distribute the color, and then activated under the dryer.

Chunking. Basically, this is similar to painting, but the lightened hair is usually kept around the face—the result is like having your own private lighting director everywhere you go.

Chipping. This technique—where only the tips of the hair are light blonde—works great with very short hairdos that can be made to stand straight up with pomade.

I'd Rather Do It Myself

You've decided that, yes, you'd like to color your hair, but you have neither the time nor the money to spend having it done professionally. So you take yourself to the drugstore and stand in the aisle in front of row after row of boxes showing photos of attractive women, each with a different hair color. These women are perfectly coifed and their message is: Use this product and maybe, just maybe, you will look like me.

Pay no attention to the front of the box. These are models with computer-assisted hair color. To choose the right color for you, check the side of the box for proper color charts.

For your first time, select something in a wash-in product close to your natural color. With this type of product, you can go a few notches darker or brighter but not lighter. If you want a radical change from brunette to blonde, the process is much more complicated, requiring peroxide and ammonia. You shouldn't attempt an extreme color change without the help of a salon professional.

If you're going to modify your color yourself, then be prepared to do it right. If the package directions indicate you should take a strand test—going through the entire process on a sample of your hair—then be sure to do it. You don't want your hair to look awful, not even for the few weeks it will take for the stuff to wash or wear away.

Simple Steps to Coloring Your Hair at Home

1. Start with a strand test, probably the most important thing you can do before you color. Select a section of hair from underneath at the back of your head or behind your ear and complete the entire coloring process on it according to the package directions. Study the results carefully. You may hate what the color has done to your hair, or you may love it. Continue if you like the color.
2. Follow the package directions to the letter. No free-styling here. Brands differ in development time; no two of them are alike.

③ Have all of your supplies within easy reach, including plastic gloves, a rattail comb, a portable clock, a hand mirror, and a second package of the product. (If you have very long hair, one package won't be enough.)

④ Protect the skin around your hairline with a thin layer of Vaseline or hair conditioner. This will keep the dye from staining your skin.

⑤ Burn incense or light a fragrance candle. The dye may have an odor that could linger in your bathroom.

⑥ Never use dye over hair that has been treated with permanent-wave solution or straighteners. This is particularly important for African American women who straighten their hair with lye solution. African American hair can be very fragile, particularly if it is curly. Each point at which the hair shaft bends is intrinsically weak, and any kind of processing, whether relaxing it with lye or permanent solutions or coloring it with a peroxide product, will damage the hair more. This is why colorists will refuse to tint or dye African American hair that has just been relaxed. Chances are, if you are an African American woman with blonde hair, it's either very short or it's artifically extended. Overprocessed hair looks fried, strawlike, dry, and damaged. Only a very short haircut can cure such damage.

⑦ Start by coloring your roots. The dye will take better closer to the warmth of your scalp. Use your fingers to broadcast the color up and through your hair. Be sure to use gloves, because the dye will stain your skin and will have to wear off.

⑧ When the color has taken, be sure to rinse it out of your hair carefully, keeping it out of your eyes. If you're using your kitchen or bathroom sink, keep a towel handy. If you are rinsing it off in the shower, don't bend your head so the dye will get in your eyes.

9. Style your hair as usual. Do you like the color? Keep a hair-dye diary for future reference, logging the product name, what you did, and how long it took you to do it.
10. Be alert to any allergic reaction. If your scalp starts to itch, break out, or bother you at all once you've distributed the dye over it (this may show up as early as the strand test) discontinue use immediately.

How to Keep Your Color Longer

Color fades when it is exposed to sun and air. Sunshine will allow the structure of the hair to break down as color molecules degrade and oxidize. Protect any processed hair from the sun—whether it has been tinted with a temporary color or fully bleached—by wearing a hat. There is no other effective sunscreen for the hair.

Augment your new color by using a color-infused shampoo once a week. Do not use colored shampoos more often, because they will deposit more color on your hair, particularly the ends, and make it appear muddy and dull. Don't use regular shampoo too often. If you are used to washing your hair every day, don't. The shampoo can strip the toner from your hair. Use a conditioner every day to soften and protect your hair from the effects of blow-dryers, rollers, and curling irons.

Beauty Tip 24: It is better to have color done over dirty hair; the natural oils of your scalp will protect it and keep it from becoming irritated.

What Causes Damaged Hair and What Can I Do about It?

- **Split ends.** Damage at the very end of the hair shafts results in split ends. The only solution: Cut them off.
- **Frizzies.** Frizzies happen when the cuticle of the hair is disturbed by overprocessing (like using perms and tints at the same time), by friction (teasing and brushing), and by heat (blow-drying, hot rollers, curling irons), which is the biggest culprit. Friction, by the way, can be something as gentle as towel-drying your hair or simply running your fingers through it. There are anti-frizz products (heavy-duty conditioners) on the market to smooth disturbed cuticles. But the best

way to get rid of the frizzies is to avoid them altogether. Be gentle with your hair; do not snap combs or brushes through it; don't overprocess it; don't attempt to comb or brush wet hair without a detangler.

- **Environmental damage.** Sunlight, pollution, swimming-pool chlorine, and tap water can all dry hair. Protect your hair when you swim by rubbing in conditioner and leaving it in and by wearing a bathing cap. Rinse your hair thoroughly when you get out of the pool to get rid of chlorine. If your tap water is hard, buy shampoos and conditioners specially formulated to compensate.
- **Chemical processing.** Permanent waves, straightening, and dyes can all dry the hair and disturb the cuticle. Avoid doing two or more at the same time.

TEXTURAL CHANGE

Did you know that permanent-wave solution and straightener are almost chemically identical? The only difference in the result is how you use them—with tight little rods to impart curl to straight hair, or with weights to flatten and straighten out frizzy or curly hair. To change the natural shape of the hair shaft, the disulfide bonds in the cortex must be broken, modified, and then put back together again. That means that both processes work on the same principle: using ammonia to lift the cuticle so the wave or straightening solution can react chemically with the disulfide bonds. The chemical solution is then rinsed off with the help of a neutralizer that stops the chemical's action and causes the hair's sulfur bonds to relink in the new configuration: curled or straight.

If your hair will not stand up to an ammonia-based straightening product, your only alternative is to use a relaxer. You can find hair relaxers in two formulas—lye and no lye. The active ingredient in lye is sodium hydroxide, which breaks down the cuticle layer of the hair, allowing it to stay flat. The longer you keep the relaxer on the hair, the better it works. But the downside is that your hair becomes much more susceptible to damage.

Depending upon hair growth, chemically processed curled or relaxed hair will revert back to its natural state in two to three months. Because you've manipulated your hair's chemical makeup, it is in a fairly weakened state, which is why you should treat your hair with gentleness and respect. Permed or relaxed hair will break easily. And if you color your hair when it has been chemically treated, you're asking for trouble.

Waving Goodbye to Straight Hair

How many of us have survived the home permanent? I almost didn't. When I was about 9, my mother decided she wanted my fine, naturally wavy hair to be curlier, and she subjected me to a rather primitive new invention called the home permanent. Every time I use an ammonia product on my kitchen floor, memories come flooding back of our little yellow and blue tiled bathroom, suffused with toxic fumes. And I was in the middle of it, my little head crowned with tightly rolled permanent-wave rods. Did I mention I hated the results?

Although today's home permanents are technically far superior, perming at home is not something I would recommend, particularly as there are so many things a good stylist can do with your hair using specific types of professional permanent waves. Modern permanent waves are designed to create tight or loose curls, spiral curls, and flowing waves, and they add body to limp, straight hair.

The Body or Root Perm. A body perm affects the entire hair shaft, imparting a subtle wave to add more body or to change the overall shape of your hair. A root perm treats the roots of your hair and is used to create curl or body directly where your hair is the flattest. Both types of permanents add volume to the hair and make it look thicker.

Spot Perms. Used to touch up specific areas, the spot perm can add height or even out texture where the hair is straight in one place and wavier in another.

THE KINDEST CUT

It's time. That long hair you've been messing with since your college days doesn't fit you or your lifestyle anymore. You're not a kid; you've got a career. Or you're just sick of fussing. Or for years you've been washing and setting your hair yourself, and you've grown tired of it. It's time for a change. You need to see a haircutter.

If you're new in a city, it could take weeks of careful homework or a clutch of free consultations before you find a new stylist. Always, I mean *always*, take advantage of this salon service: Make an appointment with a cutter. Just to talk. A stylist acquaintance of mine calls it "the first date." Learn what he or she can offer you. If a hairdresser wants to charge you for just talking for 10 or 15 minutes, then find another.

A good stylist is an excellent questioner and an even better listener. But if you ever find yourself in the chair of a hairdresser who thinks he or she knows what is best for you, leave. Fast. Because the stylist has a specific picture in mind that may not at all resemble the picture you have.

Relationships between stylists and clients are based on trust and expectation. You trust *them* to not butcher your hair and give you a style that you're not expecting, and they trust *you* to communicate your pleasure and displeasure about what they've done. Take the time to build a relationship with someone who will respect your needs and your desires. To get to that point, your stylist should know some very important things about you, which only you can reveal:

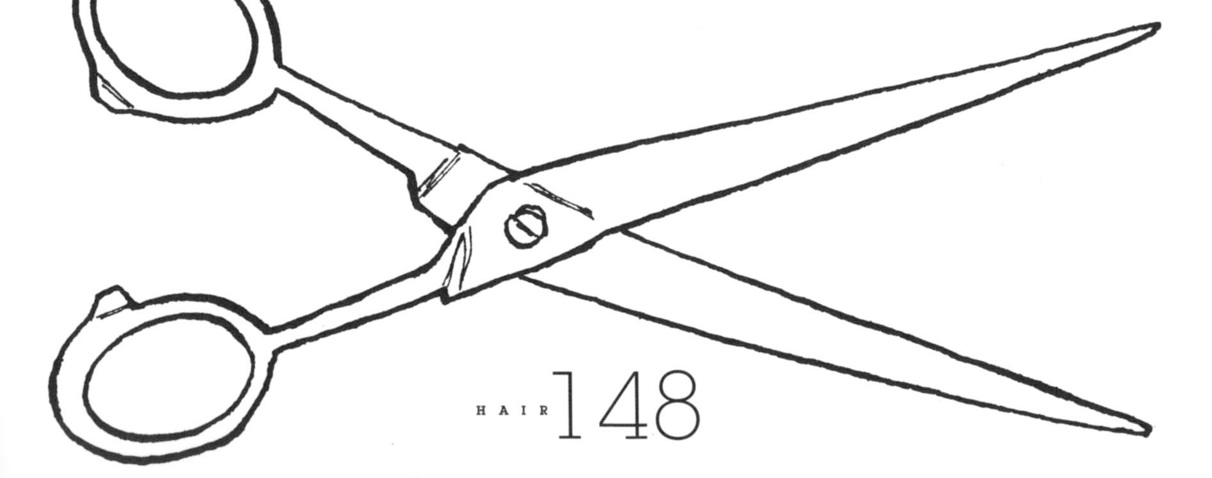

- ***Are you a homemaker and a mother, a professional woman, or a student? In other words: How much time are you going to be able to devote to fussing with your hair?***
- ***Do you like sports? Do you swim? Play tennis? Lift weights? Are you exercising and sweating so that you wash your hair daily?***
- ***Do you travel a lot? Is your hair exposed to airplane air and strange city water?***
- ***Do you want to make a drastic change? A slight change? No change at all?***
- ***Do you have a specific image you want to project? Are you a fashion person? Do you think of yourself as an outdoor person? Will your haircut have to do double-duty in your day job and your evening engagements?***
- ***How much time and money are you willing to devote to maintaining your style?***

A good haircut will balance your facial features. A good cutter will seat you straight in the chair with your legs uncrossed and will judge your positive features. A good haircut will emphasize them. At some point, you will have to acknowledge the elements of your face that are not flattering—for instance, a prominent jawbone, à la Maria Shriver, or a long, narrow face like Cher's. If you crave a severe, middle-parted straight hairdo with a square-jawed, long face—much like Angelica Huston—do you have the aplomb, personality, and high style to carry it off? If not, don't attempt it.

A skillful, perceptive cutter—part sculptor and part psychologist—will look at your bone structure, the width of your eyes, the shape of your brows, the height of your forehead, the line of your jaw, and the size of your nose before suggesting a style for you. And if you have brought a picture of what you'd like to have, ideally, the skillful, perceptive cutter will try to explain to you with a great deal of tact, why your hair will not behave as the tresses in the photo do. Or, he or she may be able to approximate the desired cut within the limitations of your hair.

Beauty Tip 25:

Arrive at the salon a bit early for a consultation with a new hairdresser so you can observe how he or she works. Is the stylist too flamboyant? Are the hairstyles too avant-garde for your taste? Does the hairdresser take too much time? If the work style does not please you, don't make an appointment.

Rule of Thumb:

The softer the brush or comb, the less damage it will do. Combs with rough teeth, brushes with hard bristles, and rubber bands will break the cuticle.

Basic Face Shapes

The object of a good haircut is to balance facial features in a symmetrical way. If you've been blessed with an oval face with regular features (which is what makes most photographic models so beautifully malleable), it won't be difficult. But not every woman's face shape is the photographer's ideal. Women's faces can be oval, elongated, round, square, or heart shaped.

The Oval Face. An oval face has the most options. You can wear your hair short, long, up, or down without changing the symmetry of your face. If your cheekbones are strong and your eyes are mesmerizing, then the haircut should focus on them. If your forehead is too high, bangs are a nice way to decrease the look of a narrower, longer oval face

The Long Face. A long face needs fullness at the sides above the chin. To complement a long face and give it attractive symmetry, the cutter will create the illusion of width to balance the length of the face. Layering around the face, especially at the cheekbone and eye area, will break up the strong vertical lines; a single-length, straight hairdo will accentuate and elongate an already long face. Bangs are a good way to shorten the face, as is a side part, which allows more volume on the sides of the face. Parting the hair to one side also adds roundness.

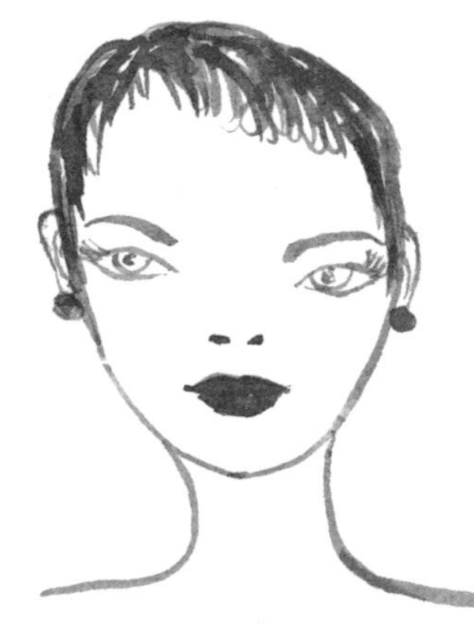

oval

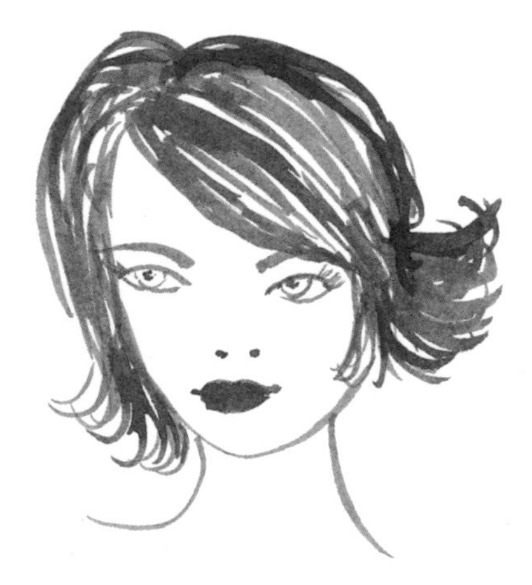

long

The Round Face. Chubby cheeks are adorable on babies, but can be a problem for a woman. The hair needs fullness at the top of the head to make the face appear longer. Any kind of geometric precision cut will accentuate the roundness. A banged bob is not the most flattering cut. One-length longer cuts work better than bobs.

The Heart-Shaped or Triangular Face. Usually, in this sweetheart shape, the cheekbones and eyes are wide, and the face tapers to a narrow chin. To de-emphasize both, hair should be full along the chin line to fill in the area so the cheeks will not dominate. The simplest cut is the inverted triangle with hair that falls long with no bangs and curves gently inward at the chin. A shorter, curly style will soften a severe appearance.

The Square Face. A square face has a strong jaw and a wide forehead and, without the proper cut, can appear hard-edged and slightly masculine. Your hairstyle should avoid emphasizing the squarest regions of your face. Layering around the face softens the lines and curly or wavy styles give the face some feminine roundness. The length of the hair should extend below the jawline. Pulled-back hairstyles serve only to shift the focus to the jawline.

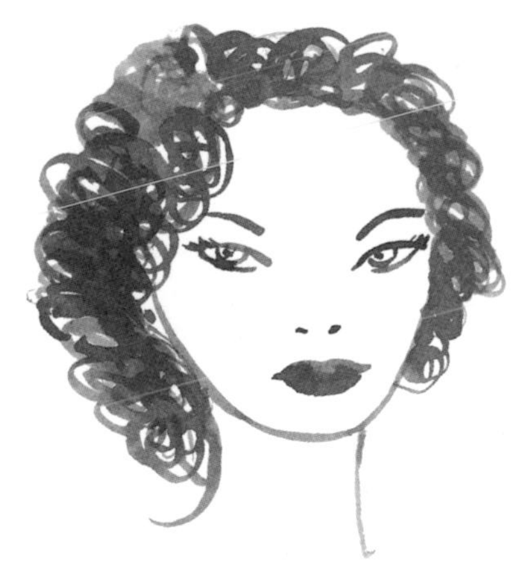

round

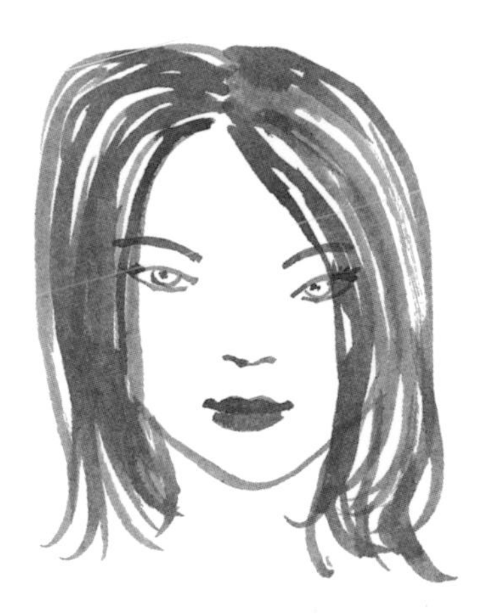

heart-shaped

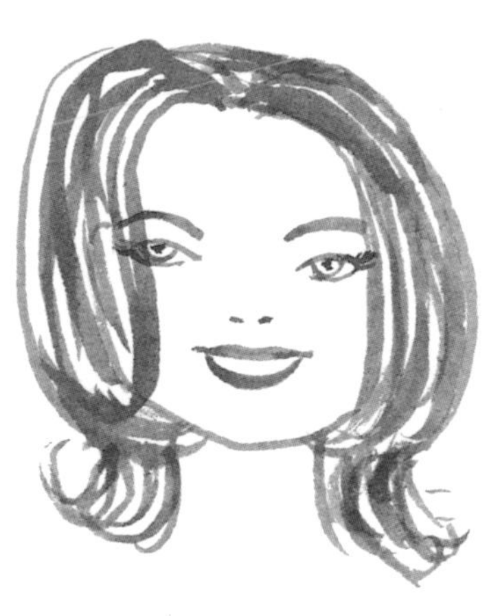

square

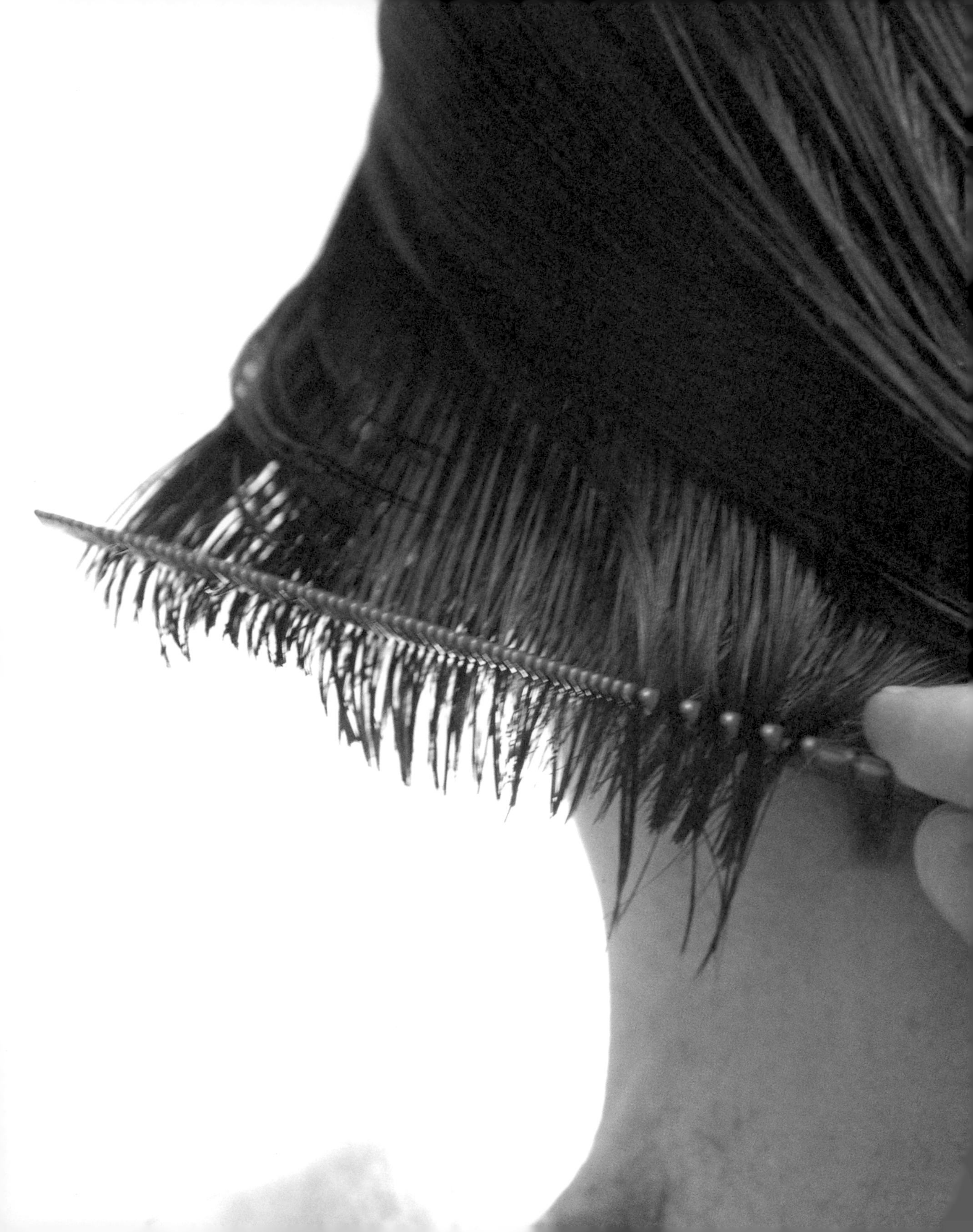

HAIR: THE RENEWABLE RESOURCE

There was once an apocryphal story about the late Sal Mineo who starred with James Dean in *Rebel without a Cause.* It was rumored that if he had a bad haircut, he would go to bed for a couple of weeks until it grew out. Most of us do not have that option. But hair, like Pinocchio's nose, does keep growing. Hair has a very tenuous life as it sprouts through our scalps. A bad haircut is the least amount of damage we can do to it.

Everything you do to your hair—from frying it with a bad perm or bleach to simply running your hands through it—has its consequences. You can dry it out, fracture the cuticle, split its ends, or turn it dull, lank, and greasy. But there are steps you can take to ensure the integrity of your hair.

- **Brushing.** Brush or comb your hair as gently as possible, using a soft brush with well-spaced bristles. Forget the 100-strokes-a-night rule; that only inflicts unnecessary damage on your hair. Instead, brush your hair gently, starting at your scalp. If you have fuller, longer hair, brush it in sections. Be careful not to snap your brush or comb through the ends of your hair. Avoid using a hairbrush on wet hair; wide-toothed combs with rounded tips have been designed for that.
- **Shampooing.** To avoid damaging the hair shaft while you're removing excess oil (sebum) and dead skin cells from your scalp, shampoo your hair close to the scalp. Massage gently (the operative word here) with your fingertips, or use your fingernails to *gently* scratch your head; this increases exfoliation of dead skin cells and blood circulation, which nourishes the hair follicles.

- **Drying.** Don't rub, wring, tousle, or twist your hair dry. With a towel, gently squeeze out the excess moisture.
- **Handling.** Be sparing in your attentions. Handle your hair as little as possible. If you have an unconscious habit of running your hands through your hair or tossing it away from your face, chances are you're disturbing the cuticle.
- **Perming and Coloring.** Do not perm and color your hair at the same time. Nothing will damage your hair more than inflicting two chemical processes on it. It's very simple. If you've seen women with dull, flyaway, dry, and lifeless hair, chances are they've tried to dye it after they've permed it. The results are not pretty.
- **Tinting/Dyeing.** Any time you change the color of your hair, you manipulate the hair's natural chemistry. Overcoloring with harsh chemicals will dry the hair; platinum-blonde hair, which requires a touch-up every two to three weeks, can look dry and damaged if it is allowed to grow long.
- **Heat.** Avoid using a hair dryer too close. Heat is your hair's natural enemy. The cuticle will shatter if you hold a hot hair dryer closer than 3 to 6 inches. Using heat usually means you want to straighten your hair using a very large, round brush, or establish curl with rollers or smaller brushes. But if you subject your hair to too much heat—too much blow-drying or blow-drying with high heat settings—then no product will be able to fix the damage.

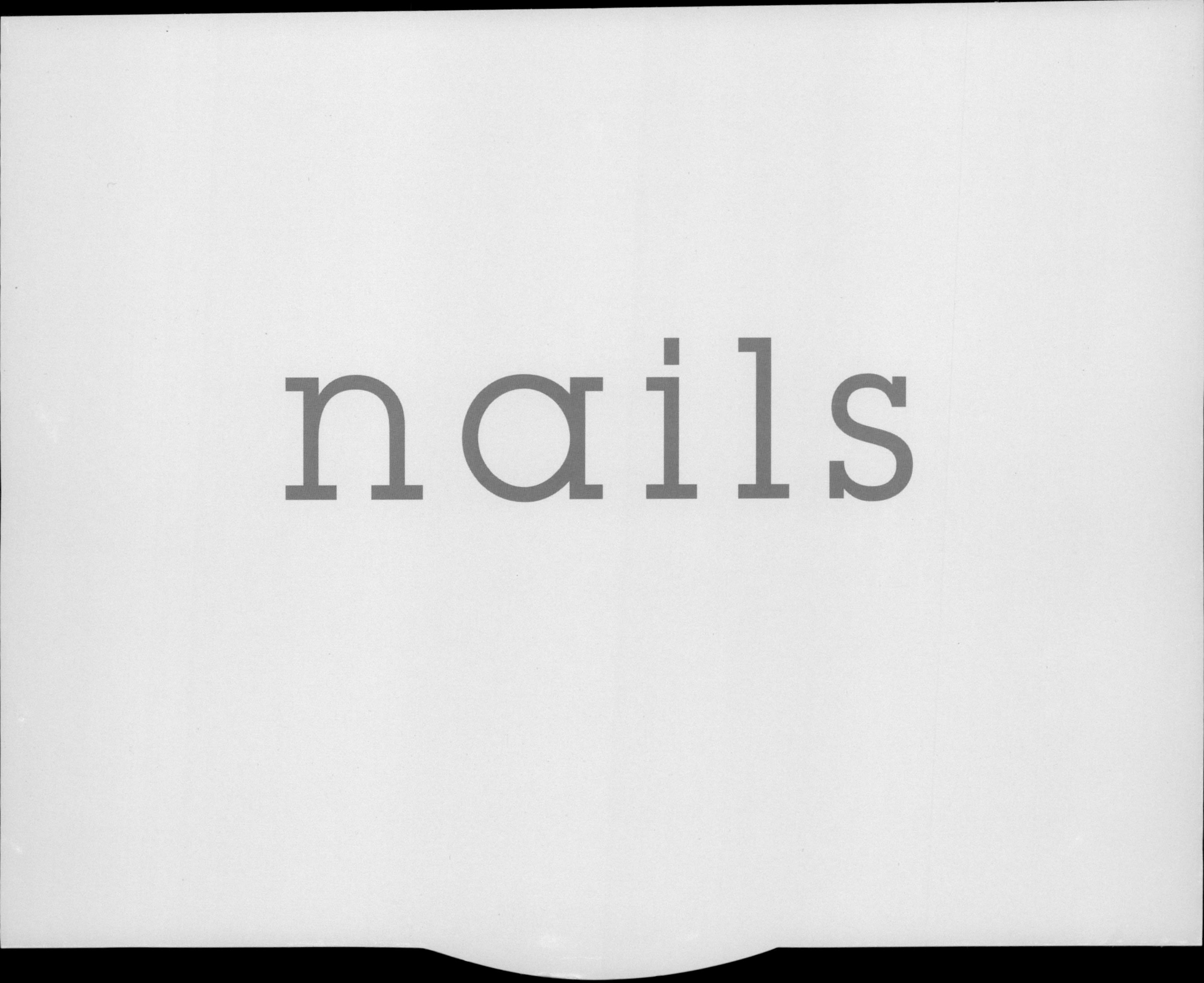
nails

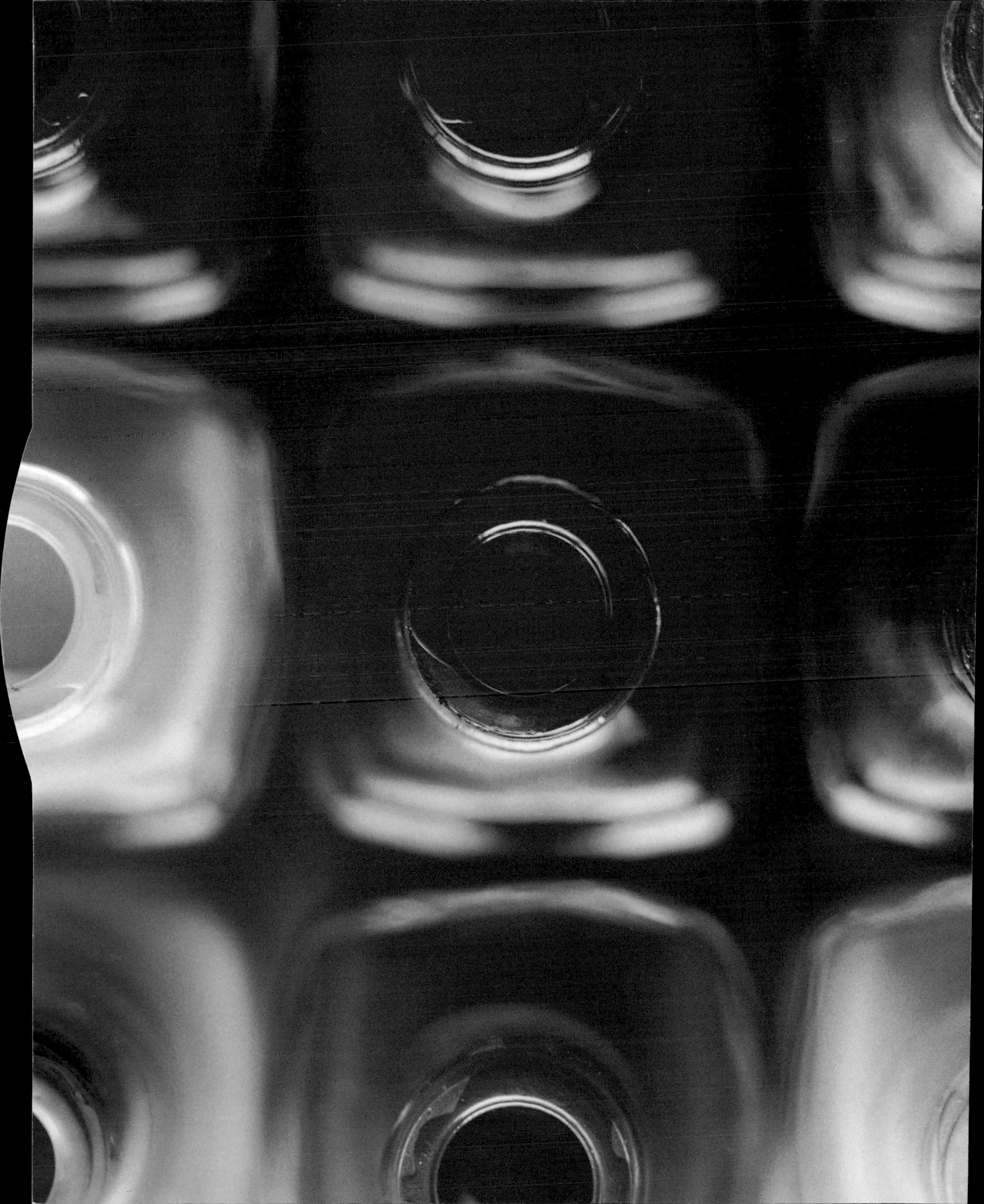

CHAPTER FIVE: NAILS

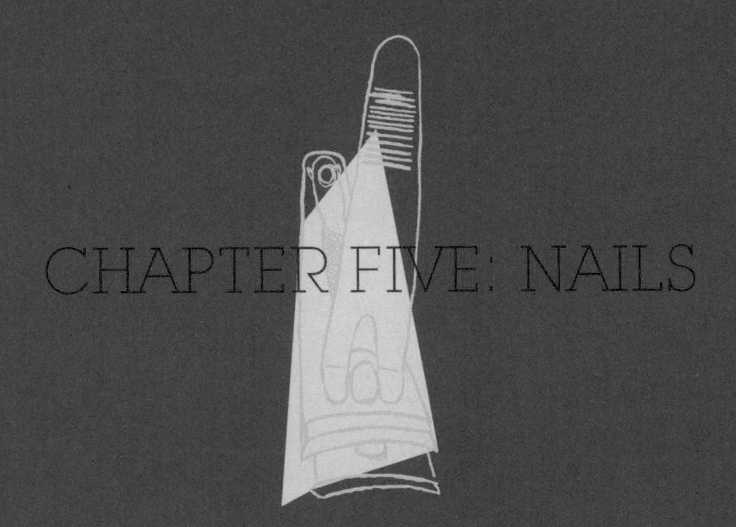

Hands can reveal a woman's age, her economic status, occupation, hobbies, and inner torments.

Nothing says more about a woman's age and temperament than her hands and nails. She could be clothed by the finest designers; her face could be a miracle of the plastic surgeon's art, and her skin could be as unblemished and smooth as marble—all this possible with today's modern cosmetic and surgical techniques. But her hands and nails will never lie.

Hands can reveal a woman's age, her economic status, occupation, hobbies, and inner torments. With their telltale freckles, age spots, and rough, torn nails, hands will reveal that what looks like a society woman, a finely wrought beauty, loves the feel of the earth under her hands—gardening without gloves. Hands will tell that a woman plays golf (the glove-wearing hand will be paler than the other hand) or tennis (calluses on the palm) or that she types into a computer (short nails). And a perfect manicure might be the sign of self-pampering: a routine that takes her from spa to salon to luncheon. If her nails are bitten to the quick, or if a thumb is ragged with hangnails, her hands may reveal a stressful life.

Our hands are instruments of expression. How many of us couldn't talk without using them? And how many of us sit on our hands, bury them deeply in pockets, or keep them shoved under the table because we're ashamed of how they look? Unless we wear gloves during all of our waking hours, our hands are a dead giveaway, blabbing secrets our lips would never tell.

It does not have to be that way. With the right kind of care—beginning with neat, clean nails and cream-softened skin—hands have the potential for charm and seduction, right in their graceful palms. Because they are our most expressive appendages, they deserve to be well cared for, cosseted, protected, and accented by beautiful, healthy nails.

NAIL NUTRITION

The nutritional rules that apply to a healthy body apply to healthy nails. They're all part of the same package. Your nails, like every cell structure of your body, are made of keratin—the same form of protein that creates feathers on birds, scales on fish, hoofs on horses, and the hair on your head. But

what you eat, as well as your general health, can affect the strength, appearance, and health of your nails.

Your body may be able to take a fad or crash diet, but chances are, your hair, skin, and nails can't. Nutritional deficiencies show up as dry skin and listless, dull hair—and as weak, fragile, splitting, misshapen nails. There is no miracle cure; only sensible eating, which includes those recommended vitamins and minerals that promote excellent general health—vitamins A, B-complex, C, and E; calcium, iron, and zinc; protein from fish, eggs, meat, legumes, and dairy foods—will help.

NAIL ANATOMY

Nails mirror the body's general health, as does your skin. Were your body in optimum shape, the ideal and normal nail would be firm, flexible, slightly pink in color, with a smooth, curved, unspotted surface free of ridges and craters. Nature made nails to protect the tips of our fingers and toes. What we see sitting at the end of each finger is not only dead keratin, but also the exposed end of a complicated network of cell-producing areas, blood vessels, and nerves. Examine your own forefinger; compare it to the diagram and the following description:

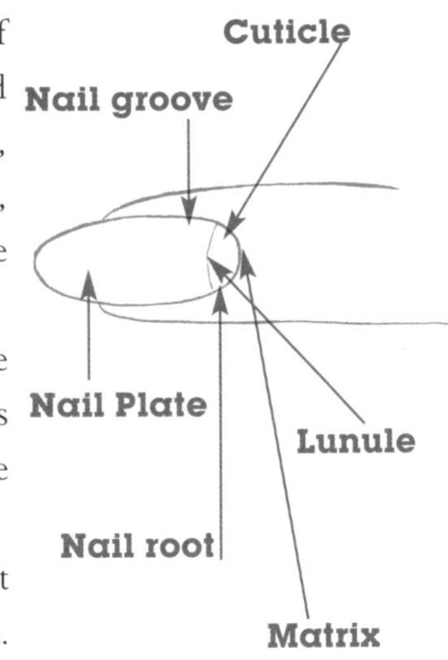

- **Nail Body or Nail Plate.** This is the visible portion of the nail, attached to the delicate nail bed beneath it. The nail body extends from the root of the nail to what manicurists call the free edge, where the nail ends at the tip of the finger.
- **Nail Bed.** The portion of skin upon which the nail plate rests. It starts in the matrix at the base of the nail and ends before the free edge. Like skin, it is made up of different layers, the dermis and the epidermis. The epidermis, connected to the underside of the nail plate, moves with the nail. It has blood vessels and nerves and provides water, oxygen, and nutrients for the continued growth of the nail.
- **Matrix.** The most important part of the nail, the matrix, is located in the area of the nail bed that extends beneath the root; it is the

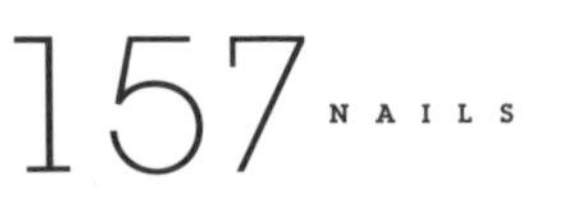

source of all new nail cells and contains nerves and lymph and blood vessels. The matrix will continue to grow fresh nail cells as long as it receives nutrition and stays healthy.

- **Nail Root.** The base of the nail, which originates in the matrix.
- **Nail Mantle.** The skin of the finger that protects the nail root.
- **Nail Groove.** The tracks on either side of the nail plate, which hold the plate in place on top of the finger.
- **Cuticle.** The overlapping tight skin around the base of the nail.
- **Lunule.** The crescent-shaped area peeking out from the cuticle where the matrix and nail bed join; not all nails have a visible lunule. It determines the shape of the nail plate and echoes the shape of the free edge.

A PROFESSIONAL MANICURE

One of life's greatest pleasures is the kind of pampering an excellent manicurist can provide when she or he does the nails on your hands or gives you a pedicure. From the first swish of pungent nail-polish remover, manicures are one of my favorite indulgences. Pedicures, especially if the manicurist gives a great foot massage, can put me into orbit.

But for the first-timer, manicures and pedicures can be fairly intimidating experiences. Before you step into your neighborhood nail parlor or make an appointment at a busy, downtown salon, assess the skills of the manicurist. Here is a checklist for you. A good manicurist:

- Understands the structure of the hands, arms, and nails.
- Works easily with his or her tools.
- Works on your nails quickly, efficiently, deftly, painlessly (relatively), and with a minimum of conversation.
- Improves your nails.

- Should have beautiful, or at least well-kept, nails herself.
- Has sanitary equipment.
- Will be licensed, and so will the salon.
- Will not use illegal tools on your hands or feet (such as implements with sharp razor blades for cutting calluses, which are outlawed in New York, California, and numerous other states).
- Will provide a wide selection of polish colors.
- Will use your own nail polish if you prefer and will hold it for you for future visits.

There are many reasons to have a professional manicure, but the main one is to inspire you to take better care of your hands. When you know that you're paying to have your nails shaped, your cuticles neatened, your hangnails tended, and your nails buffed or polished, you'll be less likely to put your hands in harm's way. For nail biters especially, having professional manicures—in fact, booking a standing appointment every week—might be the only way you'll ever quit biting. (It worked for me.)

Rule of Thumb:

Dark nail polish is high maintenance; it requires constant attention. Lighter polishes do not show wear as readily and don't look quite as unsightly if they chip.

I'D RATHER DO IT MYSELF

For whatever reason—whether a matter of money, time, or the availability of a reputable salon—you'd prefer to do your nails yourself. There is something incredibly peaceful (not to mention feminine) about doing your own nails. It can bring up fond memories of Mama painting your tiny nails with bright pink polish when you were 4, or those sleepovers with friends where everyone ended up with some glittery, violet nail polish purchased that afternoon at the drugstore.

Add a weekly manicure to your special at home indulgence evening. Plan to give your nails a treat and a treatment at least once a week.

The Toolbox

Although it would be lovely if a friend gifted you with a nifty little manicure kit, chances are it would not contain enough of the right tools to do you much good. The best approach is to go to a beauty supply store and stock up on nail products and manicure tools. Here's what you'll need:

Brush. Excellent for cleaning nails after you've been gardening, painting, or working with dust or dirt. Try using a toothbrush; it is not as rough as a nailbrush.

Buffer (Handheld). A piece of chamois or leather attached to a plastic handle. Sweep it in one direction, away from base of nail (scrubbing it back and forth can cause burning, and the nail can dry out with overbuffing).

Buffer (Stick Version). This implement looks like an oversized emery board with rounded edges. You can buy one in varying grades of abrasiveness to buff ridges on top of nails; use the softest grade to gently smooth the nail, which increases blood circulation in the nail bed.

Buffing Disk. Usually made with finer grades of sandpaper, a buffing disk is used to smooth any rough nail edges or to buff the surface of the nail to soften ridges.

Clippers. Handy for shortening extra-long nails; a larger size is used for pedicures.

Cuticle Nippers. Clips away loose skin around the cuticle (but never for cutting the cuticle itself). Do not use these nippers for cutting nails; it will dull the blades.

Emery Board. For shortening and shaping nails, this disposable, long, flexible cardboard implement usually has two sides, with coarse emery on one side and fine emery on the other. The coarse side is for radically reducing the size of the nail; the fine side is for refining the free edge.

Foot Scraper. This paddle with an abrasive oval is used to reduce calluses and to remove dead skin from the bottom and sides of your feet.

Orange Stick. Made of orangewood or plastic, an orange stick is used to push the cuticles back (gently, please) and remove dirt from under

the nail. Also can be used to correct polish mistakes when wrapped in a thin layer of cotton dipped in remover.

Polish-Remover Pad. Make sure the pad is lint free, so cotton residue will not remain on nails when you remove your polish.

Nail Scissors. Can be used for cutting silk or paper for nail wraps or for trimming hangnails; please don't use them for cutting cuticles.

Pumice Stone. Used in pedicures, a pumice stone removes hardened patches of skin on the foot.

Toenail/Fingernail Cutters. Resembling clippers but larger and stronger, these cutters can be used to cut toenails or to clip the sides of toenails to prevent ingrown nails.

Toe Separator. A rubber form that is placed between toes, before application of polish, to keep toes from touching each other (or, you can use a piece of tissue—twisted and woven through your toes).

White Pencil. Use to whiten the underside of the nail—for a French manicure or when buffing your nails; also handy for drawing a guideline for a French manicure.

Nail-Care Products

Professional manicurists have entire workstations full of tools at their fingertips to make sure yours are groomed and polished up prettily. With beauty supply and drug stores stocked with basically the same kinds of products, you can purchase nail polish, topcoats, base coats, fortifiers, ridge fillers, glitter, and decals for doing your nails at home. The basic kit should include:

Polish Remover. This pungent liquid solvent removes nail polish and is available in different formulas: with acetone for removing polish from natural nails and without acetone for removing polish from acrylics or fake nails.

Cuticle Oil. This lubricates the cuticle and keeps it soft and healthy; it can be used at bedtime or during a manicure to help soften the cuticle so it can easily be pushed back with a towel or an orange stick.

Modern polish has been around since the 1920s, and though there have been many improvements—such as quick-drying, one-step, metallic, and sheer varieties—the formula is still based on a combination of four ingredients.

These are

- polymers like nitrocellulose or TSF resin, which improve adhesion and toughen the polish.
- plasticizer to increase flexibility and wear (usually in the form of castor oil).
- solvents such as toluene, ethyl alcohol, or ethyl acetate for spreadability.
- pigments, which provide color and coverage.

Cuticle Cream. Used to remove dead skin around the cuticle.

Liquid Wrap Fluid or Silk Wrap Material. For temporary repairs on breaks and tears or to strengthen weak nails, wraps are used in conjunction with nail glue or superglue.

Ridge Filler. This form of base coat evens out ridges, gullies, and lines on nails; it can be used either under a regular base coat or as base coat itself.

Nail Hardener. This nail treatment strengthens weak nails.

Base Coat. This primer coat may look cloudy in the bottle, but it dries clear, smoothes out the top of the nail, and leaves a slightly tacky surface, so nail polish will go on evenly and adhere better.

Nail Polish. Also called nail enamel and nail lacquer, Europeans refer to it as nail varnish. Modern nail polish is available in many textures, hues, and degrees of sheerness including, from the least amount of color to the most: sheer, stain, shimmer, metallic, frost, cream, and matte.

Topcoat. This clear finish dries transparent and helps increase the life of the manicure.

Decals. These teensy cut-out designs come in any number of imaginative forms, from stars, moons, and comets to cartoon characters and astrological signs for decorating nails.

Sealer. Denser and more viscous than topcoat, a sealer protects decals and other painted nail decor.

Nail Evaluation

Before you take an emery board or nail file to your nails, look at your hands. Ask yourself some basic questions about your nails and your lifestyle:

- **Are my fingers long or short? Tapered or pudgy?**
- **What shape are my fingernails: oval, square, fan, arched, flat, angular, narrow, wide, concave, or convex?**
- **Are my nails ridged, broken, bitten, or striated with white lines?**
- **Are my cuticles ragged, bitten, split, tight?**

- **What kind of lifestyle do I have? Are my hands in water often? Do I use a computer? Do I like crafts, gardening, sports? Do I dress up a lot? Do I play an instrument?**

The answers to these questions will determine how much care your hands and nails require, the most practical length for your nails, and the limitations of what you can do with them. After you've answered the questions above, consider the following:

- **Hand Shape.** Long, tapered, graceful fingers with oval-shaped nails are such an ideal that, probably, only hand models have them. The shape you decide to make your nails should compliment your hands and fingers—usually nail form follows the shape of the cuticle at the base of the nail and is echoed in the shape of the finger at the free edge. Long talons on lengthy, tapering fingers may look dramatic and threatening, but shorter, neater, more squared-off nails would compliment and enhance long fingers.
- **Stress Level.** Your hands, as individual as your eyes, lips, hair, and skin, can reflect your diet or your stress level.
- **Damaged Nails.** If your nails are striated with white lines, ridged, pitted, split, or break easily, you might want to observe what and how you are eating. Many nail weaknesses can be improved by a diet higher in protein and calcium. For temporary relief, try nail creams, nail hardeners, or ridge fillers.
- **Bad Habits.** Your cuticles are a mirror of your lifestyle and stress level. Do you bite the sides of your thumbs when you're nervous, or pick at your cuticles when you're stopped at a red light? Do you chew hangnails unconsciously? What would it take to get you to stop chewing on your nails and cuticles? Paying attention might help. Try carrying clove or cinnamon sticks to chew on, instead of your fingers. And whenever possible, remove yourself from stressful situations.

Beauty Tip 26:
Store your polish in a cool, dry place away from heat and light.

Beauty Tip 27:
Run a white nail pencil under the free edge of the nail to make the nail edge look even whiter, especially for a French manicure.

Rules of Thumb:

Keep these points in mind when you are shaping your nails:

- **Never file wet nails. It can weaken them.**
- **For a graceful, natural nail, the shape should echo that of the shape of the cuticle around the lunule.**
- **Avoid filing deep into the corner of a nail; that weakens the nail. Besides, if the nail extends past the fingertip before it is shaped, it will appear longer.**

Basic at-Home Manicure

Once you've looked at your hands critically and have begun to be conscious of what you are doing with your hands, it's time to do your nails.

Step One. Remove old polish with a cotton pad and polish remover.

Step Two. Shape your nails. Usually, the free edge of the nail will echo the shape of your cuticle—oval, square, or rounded square. The nail should look symmetrical at the root and at the free edge. If your nails are too long, you can use a nail clipper to take off the excess and an emery board to refine the shape and smooth the rough edges. Avoid using a sawing, back and forth motion; use the emery board in one direction only, starting at the outside edge of the nail and working in. Then change direction to even up the opposite side.

Step Three. Wash your hands to rid them of solvent and dust; if you have the time, soak them in sudsy water to help soften your cuticles. (To make cuticle care even easier, you might want to give yourself a manicure after you've had a bath or a shower.)

Step Four. Rub each nail with a dab of cuticle cream or cuticle remover. To loosen the cuticle, work around it gently with the blunt edge of an orange stick. (For easier care, you can use a towel to push back your cuticles after a bath or after washing your hands; in addition, you can treat your cuticles with oil each night before you go to sleep.)

Step Five. Clean under the free edge of the nail with a cotton-tipped orange stick, soaked in water.

Step Six. Check your cuticles and take this opportunity to trim remaining hangnails and dead cuticle with cuticle clippers.

Step Seven. Refine the shape of your nails one last time with the finer side of your emery board, and wash your hands one more time, drying them completely.

Step Eight. Apply protein builder or ridge filler if needed, then the base coat.

Step Nine. Apply polish. Dip the brush into the bottle, wipe off any excess on the inside of the bottle lip, and apply quickly, starting with a stroke

down the center of the nail and adding a stroke on either side. Redip brush for each nail.

Step Ten. Apply topcoat to the nail and under the nail tip. To make your manicure last longer, reapply topcoat every two or three days.

Step Eleven. Neaten up nails by removing excess polish with an orange stick dipped into nail polish remover. Or you can wrap the orange stick with a twirl of cotton, but squeeze out excess liquid before using.

Step Twelve. Allow polish to dry for at least 15 minutes.

Nail Tips from the Pros

Here are a few tips from professional manicurists to remember when applying colored polish:

- **Shake the bottle to mix polish thoroughly.**
- **Apply polish with quick, light strokes, first at the very center of the nail and then on each side. That way, you will deposit the heaviest amount of polish in the middle of your nail where it can't run into the side grooves.**
- **Redip your brush for each nail.**
- **Always apply two coats (sometimes even a third, if polish is thin and fairly transparent).**
- **If you've gotten polish on your skin or in the nail groove, dip an orange stick into polish remover, shake off the excess, and use it to remove the offending smudge.**
- **When applying sheer polish, to prevent a striping effect, wait until the first coat has dried completely before putting on a second.**
- **When you apply polish, be patient and let it dry on its own. Slower-evaporating solvents make the color more vivid. Blowing on freshly polished nails to dry them will lower adhesion and gloss.**

Rule of Thumb:

Never, never, never cut your cuticle. It is there to protect the nail bed from damage. If you cut your cuticles, you're courting infection.

Rule of Thumb:

Avoid using the professional manicurist's metal cuticle tool at home; you can easily damage the cuticle by pressing too hard. Instead use orange sticks; they are flexible, so the potential for harm is lessened.

Beauty Tip 28:
To get the best results from your polish, use a base coat, two coats of polish, and a topcoat, and wait as long as you can after each coat to allow it to dry. Applying a second coat of polish too quickly will cause an uneven, orange-peel effect.

- **The best base coat is ridge filler.**
- **For base coats to adhere, make sure the nail surface is oil- and moisture-free.**
- **Don't polish your nail clear up to the cuticle; polish on or too near the cuticle will dry it.**

Quick Pedicure

The basic pedicure is much like the basic manicure. The only differences are the size of some of the equipment, the distance your arms have to reach, and the amount of drying time necessary for the polish to cure.

Step One. Remove old polish from toenails with solvent and cotton.

Step Two. Shape toenails by cutting long nails with toenail scissors and refining the shape with a nail file or a fairly rough emery board; the free edge of the nail should echo the shape of the toe tip, but still be slightly squared off.

Step Three. Soak your feet to soften the skin around the cuticles. The best time to do a pedicure at home is when you've just showered or bathed, and the skin around your toenails is soft and pliable.

Step Four. Apply cuticle cream to your toes, let it set, and then push the cuticles back with an orange stick. Gently.

Step Five. Use a pumice stone or a foot scraper to remove calluses and dead skin from the sides and bottoms of your feet.

Step Six. Massage an exfoliating cream over your feet, around your ankles, and up your shins to keep feet and ankles soft.

Step Seven. Rinse lotion and cuticle products from your toes; dry well.

Step Eight. Use separators to keep toes from touching. If you don't have toe separators, twist a tissue into a rope and lace it between your toes.

Step Nine. Polish toenails as you would fingernails—using a base coat, two coats of colored polish, and a topcoat.

Step Ten. Allow your toes to dry for at least 45 to 60 minutes before attempting to put on socks, stockings, or shoes.

Beauty Tip 29:
When your polish is open and exposed to the air, it will start to thicken. To thin it out, use a thinner designed for the purpose or add a drop of acetone polish remover and shake well.

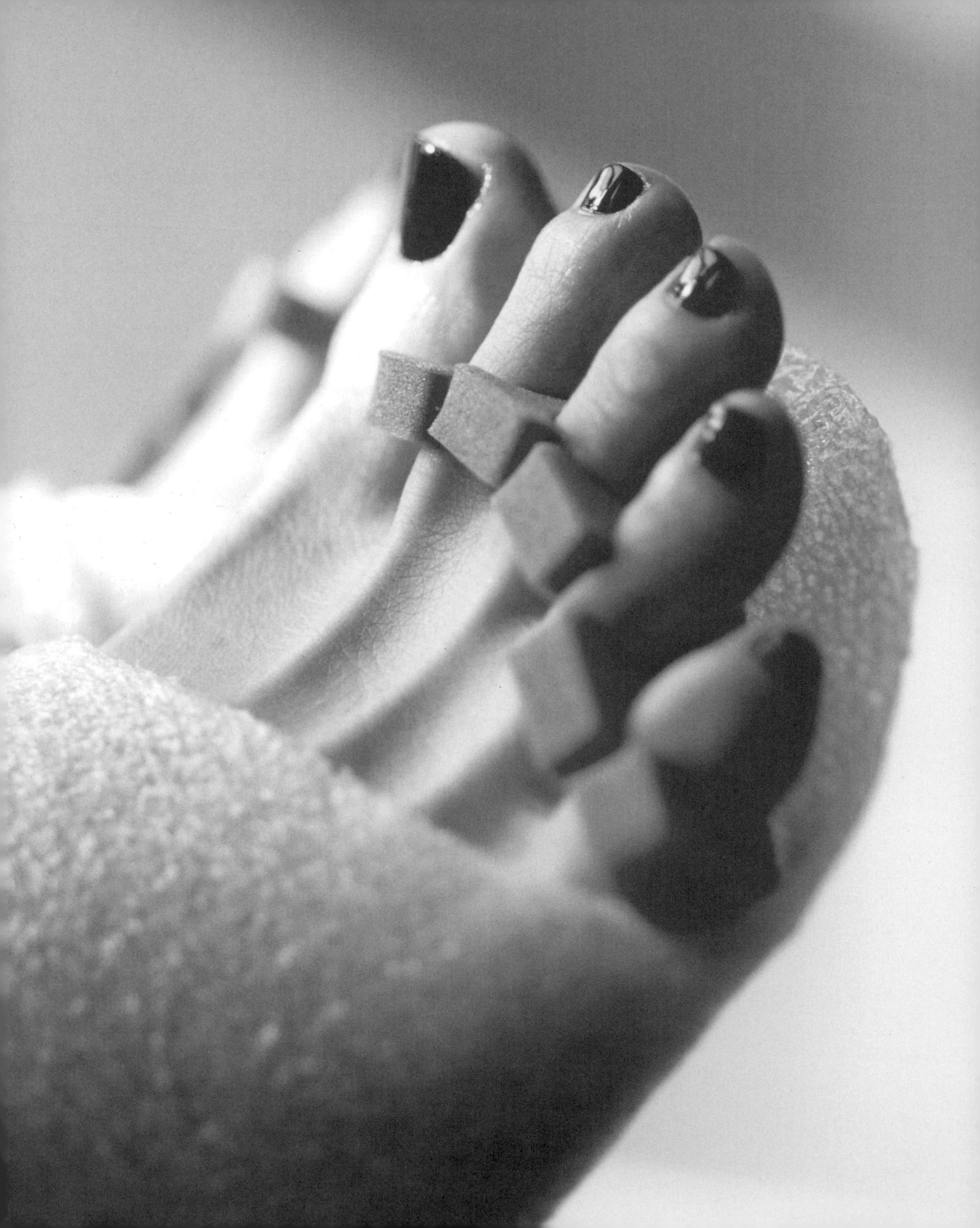

French Manicure

In the last years of the 1990s, the French manicure, on both finger- and toenails, became a popular way to wear polish that was subtle but quite fashionable. Nails did not scream out: "Look at us with bright red or flaming coral polish!" Instead, they were dressed appropriately for a boardroom or cocktail party. The look is two-toned—a light, often stark, white polish on the free edge of the nail is overlaid with two coats of pale, transparent, or translucent pink, or an off-white or a peach polish.

French manicure colors, however, could be just about anything. You're not limited to white tips—they could be off-white, cream, beige, even gold, coupled with a complementary overlay. The idea is to use two contrasting colors applied in a specific style. Let your imagination run away with you: Use dark, dark polish, something like Chanel's Vamp, and tip the nails with a metallic gold or silver.

Complete the pre-polish segment of your manicure in the usual way. Then run a white nail pencil underneath the nail; this makes the tip look whiter. Once you've primed your nails with base coat, the easiest way to accomplish the French manicure is to use Scotch tape to cover the part of the nail you don't want to paint white, then tip the nail with the opaque white or cream layer. Let the polish dry before you attempt to remove the tape. Then cover the nail with two coats of transparent polish. The new sheers that look like stained glass would be an interesting variation on the classic white tip. Always finish a French manicure the same way you would a regular one: with a high-gloss topcoat over the entire nail.

Beauty Tip 30: To prevent a French manicure from turning yellow, use a topcoat with an SPF in it. Also, avoid getting sunscreen on your nails. It will change the color of your light polish.

COMMON NAIL PROBLEMS

Wouldn't it be a perfect world if our nails never split, never broke, never got caught in car doors, never shattered or frayed? Here are the most common nail problems and what to do about them.

Beauty Tip 31: Relieve the pressure of an ingrown nail by clipping the edge of the nail; refine the edges with an emery board. If the nail is very impacted, see a podiatrist.

Broken or Split Nails. What causes them? Excessive length, carelessness, accidents, or weakness or brittleness in the nail itself. Nail oils, hardeners, and proper nutrition with calcium-rich foods can make nails stronger.

Torn Nails. Sometimes if you've let your nails grow too long or if you catch the free edge of the nail it might tear at the point where the nail emerges from the nail groove. Check first to see how far the tear extends across the nail. Chances are that you can save it by patching it with nail glue. Remove polish from the nail; squeeze a bit of nail glue (or even superglue) on the nail, and let it dry until it's tacky to the touch; then press the torn edges of the nail together. Cover the repaired nail with a piece of silk wrap cut to fit. Let it dry, then buff the nail smooth with a fine disk. Redo nail with base coat, polish, and topcoat.

BIBLIOGRAPHY

Andrews, Robert. *The Concise Columbia Dictionary of Quotations.* New York: Columbia University Press, 1990.

Angeloglou, Maggie. *A History of Makeup.* Great Britain: Macmillan, 1970.

Aucoin, Kevyn. *Making Faces.* New York: Little, Brown and Company, 1997.

——. *The Art of Makeup.* New York: Callaway Editions, 1994.

Bailey, Sheril. *The Sheril Bailey Complete Manicuring and Nail Care Handbook.* Kansas City: Andrews McMeel Publishing, 1998.

Banks, Tyra, with Vanessa Thomas Bush. *Tyra's Beauty, Inside & Out.* New York: HarperPerennial/HarperCollins, 1998.

Basten, Fred E. and Paul A. Kaufman. *Max Factor's Hollywood, Glamour, Movies, Make-Up.* Los Angeles: General Publishing Group, 1995.

Batterberry, Michael and Ariane. *Mirror Mirror, A Social History of Fashion.* New York: Holt, Rinehart and Winston, 1977.

Begoun, Paula. *Don't Go Shopping for Hair Care Products Without Me,* 2nd ed. Seattle: Beginning Press, 2000.

——. *Don't Go to the Cosmetics Counter Without Me,* 4th ed. Tukwila, WA: Beginning Press, 1998.

Broughton, Patricia, and Martha Ellen Hughes. *The Buyer's Guide to Cosmetics.* New York: Random House, 1981.

Brown, Bobbi, and Annemarie Iverson. *Bobbi Brown Beauty: The Ultimate Beauty Resource.* New York: HarperStyle/HarperCollins Publishers, 1997.

Brunas, Renato. *Renato on Color and Hair Avant-Garde.* Reading, PA: Renato Brunas, 2000.

Carr, Larry. *Four Fabulous Faces.* New York: Galahad Books, 1970.

Cimaglia, Alice R. *The Art & Science of Manicuring.* Bronx, NY: Milady Publisher Corporation, 1982.

Corson, Richard. *Fashion in Makeup, from Ancient to Modern Times.* New York: Universe Books, 1972.

Crawford, Cindy, Sonia Kashuk, and Kathleen Boyes. *Cindy Crawford's Basic Face: A Makeup Workbook.* New York: Broadway Books, 1996.

De Castlebajac, Kate. *The Face of the Century, 100 Years of Makeup and Style.* New York: Rizzoli, 1995.

Eiseman, Leatrice. *Colors for Your Every Mood: Discovering Your True Decorating Colors.* Sterling, VA: Capital Books, Inc., 1998.

Etcoff, Nancy. *Survival of the Prettiest: The Science of Beauty.* New York: Doubleday, 1999.

Falconi, Dina. *Earthly Bodies & Heavenly Hair: Natural and Healthy Personal Care for Every Body.* Woodstock, NY: Ceres Press, 1998.

Ferri, Elisa, and Lisa Kenny. *Style on Hand: Perfect Nail and Skin Care.* New York: Universe Publishing, 1998.

Garland, Madge. *The Changing Face of Beauty: Four Thousand Years of Beautiful Women*. New York: Barrows and Company, 1957.

Gross, Kim Johnson, and Jeff Stone with Rachael Urquhart. *Chic Simple: Woman's Face Skin Care and Makeup*. New York: Alfred A. Knopf, 1997.

——. *Hairdos*. New York: Stewart, Tabori & Chang, 1999.

Irons, Diane. *The World's Best-Kept Beauty Secrets*. Naperville, IL: Sourcebooks, 1997.

Jackson, Victoria, with Andrea Cagan. *Make Up Your Life: Every Woman's Guide to the Power of Makeup*. New York: Cliff Street Books/ HarperCollins Publishers, 2000.

Kehoe, Vincent Jr. *The Technique of the Professional Make-Up Artist*. Woburn, MA: Focal Press, 1995.

Leffel, David J., M.D. *Total Skin, The Definitive Guide to Whole Skin Care for Life*. New York: Hyperion, 2000.

Luscher, Max. *The Luscher Color Test*. Basel, Switzerland: Test-Verlag, 1969.

Mancuso, Kevin. *The Mane Thing*. New York: Little, Brown and Company, 1999.

Miller, Jean-Chris. *The Body Art Book, A Complete, Illustrated Guide to Tattoos, Piercings, and Other Body Modifications*. New York: Berkley Books, 1997.

Moffitt, Peggy, and William Claxton. *The Rudi Gernreich Book*. Cologne, Germany: Taschen, 1999.

Mulvey, Kate, and Melissa Richards. *Decades of Beauty: The Changing Image of Women, 1890s to 1990s*. New York: Checkmark Books, 1998.

Pallingston, Jessica. *Lipstick: A Celebration of the World's Favorite Cosmetic*. New York: St. Martin's Press, 1999.

Peters, Vicki. *M'Lady Salon Ovations' Nail Q&A Book*. Albany, NY: Milady Publishing, 1996.

Quant, Mary. *Ultimate Makeup & Beauty* London: Dorling Kindersley Limited, 1996.

Ragas, Meg Cohen, and Karen Kozlowski. *Read My Lips, A Cultural History of Lipstick*. San Francisco: Chronicle Books, 1998.

Schoon, Douglas D. *M'Lady's Nail Structure & Product Chemistry*. Albany, NY: M'Lady Publishing, 1996.

Shipman, David. *The Great Movie Stars, The Golden Years*. New York: Hill and Wang, 1970.

Simon, Diane. *Hair: Public, Political, Extremely Personal*. New York: St. Martin's Press, 2000.

Spillane, Mary, and Christine Sherlock. *Color Me Beautiful's Looking Your Best: Color, Makeup, and Style*. London: Madison Books, 1995.

Vyas, Bharti, with Claire Haggard. *Beauty Wisdom: The Secret of Looking and Feeling Fabulous*. London: Thorsons, 1997.

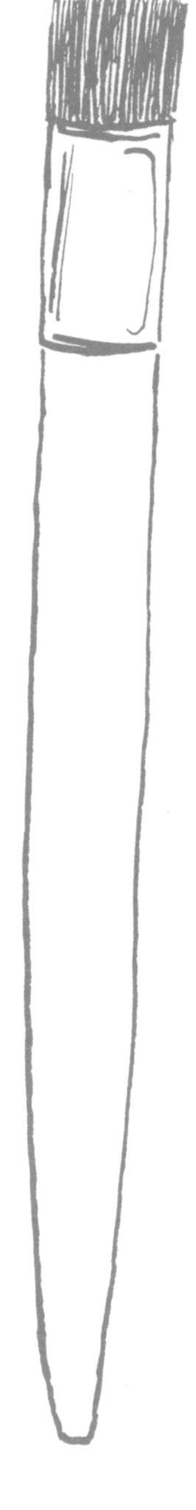

ACKNOWLEDGMENTS

In the 24 years I have been writing about beauty—skincare, makeup, hair, and nails—I have met extraordinary people who have whetted my appetite for information and knowledge. Some of them were generous enough to help me research this book: Estée Lauder's color whiz, Dominique Szabo; Chanel's charming Guy Lento; cosmetic company gurus François Nars, Laura Mercier, Vincent Longo, Trish McEvoy, Paula Dorf, Sona Kashak, and Sylvie Chantecaille; makeup artists Coreen Cordova, Joe Costa, David Starr, Tricia Saunders, Alexis Simonsen, Robyn Cosio (AKA the Eyebrow Queen), Cheryl Johns, Rocky Zion, and Robert Williams; hair gurus Frédèric Fekkai, Brad Johns, and John Barrett. A special thank you to the experts at the Vidal Sassoon Hair Academy in Santa Monica: Caroline Hays-Thomas, Stephan Moody, Sean Michael McDaniels, Julian Perlingiero, and Lucie Doughty; dermatologists Dr. Seth Matarasso and Dr. Richard Glogau; plastic surgeons Dr. Brunno Ristow, Dr. Jack Owsley, and Dr. Gerald Imber; aesthetician Angelina Umansky (who has kept my skin in tip-top shape) of Spa Radience in San Francisco; Paul Wilner, my editor at the former *San Francisco Examiner Magazine*, who agreed that beauty coverage had a place in his magazine; and Heidi Benson, former *Examiner* style editor, who encouraged thoughtful and knowledgeable beauty coverage.

I am deeply indebted to those cosmetic companies that have contributed to the color charts and photography for this book: BeneFit, Bobbi Brown, Bourjois, Calvin Klein, Chanel, Estée Lauder, François Nars, M.A.C., Stila, Vincent Longo, and Yves Saint Laurent. In addition, thank you to Jean Danielson, Jane Ford, and Arianne Damboise, BeneFit; Rosemarie Sterling and Stephanie von Stein, Chanel; Alison Mazzola, YSL; Marie-Clare Katigbak, Bobbi Brown; Shannon Cooney, Calvin Klein; Donna Italiano, Vincent Longo; Julie Leong, M.A.C.; Tiffany Carter, Estée Lauder; and Kate Sullivan, François Nars.

To color psychologist Leatrice Eiseman, author of *Colors for Your Every Mood*, I owe a huge debt for the basic information about color, its history, and its psychological and emotional meanings.

I thank attorney Bryan Rohan for bringing me my feisty agent, Maureen "The Mighty Mo" Regan, who doubles as the little sister I never had.

And last, but not least, my editor at Chronicle Books, Leslie Jonath, who brought the project to me and saw it through to the end, and her patient assistant, Jodi Davis.

CREDITS

PHOTOGRAPHER'S CREDITS

I would like to thank Julie Muszynski for her incredible eye, taste, and patience; my photo assistants, Kate Kunuth and Bert Obrentz for their steady hands; models: Kira Bronston, Erin Shaffer, Susan Felice, Sara Wolf, Suzanne A. Black, and Vicki Wright. Thank you to Daniel Freeman of Architects & Heroes; Gregory Gaston, Ashley Frost, and Kristen Nelson of Zendo Spa and Salon; Joseph Cozza and everyone at his Salon; to Julie and Aldo for the push; to Mom, Dad, Jill, Arlene, Anna, Bradley, Deborah, Lynn, Sandy, and Sheri for their support; to Carly, Olivia, and Mollie Rose for being true beauties.

Many, *many* thanks to Leslie Jonath and Jodi Davis at Chronicle Books for being so great to work with, and a special thank you to Laura Lovett for being equally wonderful and tolerating my thousands of questions; answering them with patience and insight. And most of all, thank you to Gary, Xander, and Julius for their endless inspiration.

Index